THE DIVIDING OF WOMEN or WOMAN'S LOT

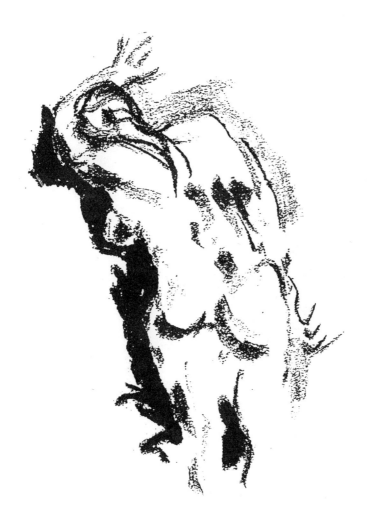

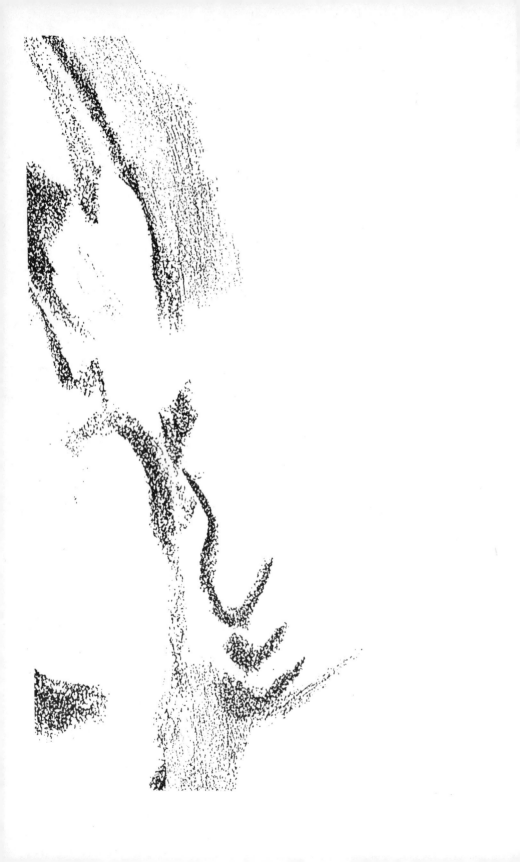

The Dividing of Women
or Woman's Lot

by

EUGÉNIE LEMOINE-LUCCIONI

Translated by Marie-Laure Davenport
and Marie-Christine Réguis

*'an association in which the free development of each
is the condition for the free development of all'*

Free Association Books / London / 1987

English language edition first published 1987 by
Free Association Books
26 Freegrove Road
London N7 9RQ

Originally published in French under the title
Partage des femmes, © Editions du Seuil 1976
Glossary © Eugénie Lemoine-Luccioni 1987

Translation © Marie-Laure Davenport and Marie-Christine Réguis 1987

The publisher gratefully acknowledges the financial assistance of the French
Ministry of Culture in defraying part of the cost of translation.

British library Cataloguing in Publication Data

Lemoine-Luccioni, Eugénie
    The dividing of women or woman's lot.
    1. Pregnancy—Psychological aspects
    I. Title   II. Partage des femmes.   *English*
    155.6'33   RG560

    ISBN 0 946960 85 2 hb
    ISBN 0 946960 86 0 pb

Typeset by Rapidset and Design Ltd, London WC1

Printed and bound in Great Britain by
Short Run Press, Exeter

CONTENTS

THE French title of this book is **Partage des femmes.**
Partage has a variety of meanings, only two of which –
'dividing' and 'lot' – have been rendered in the English title
and its extension. The extension of the title of the English
edition is an attempt to accommodate the sense of lot, which
is as immediately present to a French ear in **partage** as is the
sense of dividing. But equally the word carries the meanings
of sharing, sharing out and distributing – encompassing
both the action and the result of the action.

Another word in the French text is **partition**, which has
been translated throughout as 'division'. However, the word
is quite close to the English 'partition', again in its sense of
sharing out or dividing.

From the outset the attraction of the book resided for us
in the word **partage** and the way in which its use comes to
punctuate the text. The coincidence – and if it is one, it
certainly is no surprise – is that we, two women, shared the
translation of a book called **Partage des femmes.**

Usually a translation takes place between two people: the
author and the translator. Here, there was to be a second
layer of two people sharing the work – another division of
labour, between divided women.

We are not experts in Lacanian theory. On a first reading,
the text seduced us into believing it was quite accessible.
Accessible and rather beautiful. As the work progressed we
were compelled to review our first impression of it. We had
been sadly mistaken. We had to acknowledge with some dis-
comfort that we could make little sense of the little diagrams.
Some words escaped our understanding; sometimes whole
sentences did. Even short passages left us breathless and

troubled. When meaning was lacking for us, we held firmly to our grammar and the structure of sentences.

Strangely, this repeated experience of momentary blindness did not discourage us. Most of the text rewarded our efforts – in particular, the clinical examples, which we found profoundly illuminating for the construction of women's internal world.

The issue of sexual identity in this book is not a given, determined by gender and the capacity to bear children. The consequences of biology rather bypass the issue. Sexual identity is something to struggle with, acquire and conquer. Being a woman is hard to achieve.

We wish to thank Bernard Burgoyne for his help.

Introduction

WE shall speak of men and women here as if the distinction was self-evident. It is enough for us, indeed, that they are differentiated as being each the fantasy of the other. From that point on, it is possible to wonder in which path this fantasy takes them and how far it leads them.

In fact, it leads them, at the present time, to a crisis point. There is dispute and there is complaint—complaint in the legal sense of the term. But the reasons that are put forward are all untenable. Because, like all rationalizations, they cover and maintain an unavowed benefit; if it is true that no one can nor should accept slavery, the only question which remains when it is accepted, even requested, is this: What is it accepted for, for what benefit?

Nevertheless, it is not possible not to hear this complaint. And if the reasons put forward by women are not very convincing, it is, however, necessary to take note of their violence as a reason, against the violence to which they are subjected. A complaint for ever set in the mythical world, and which is reduced to these words which are screamed and spewed out by Marie Cardinal in the account she gives of her analysis (1973).

*If I could have known the harm she (my mother) was going to do to me, if . . . I could have imagined the **ugly, incurable** wound that she was going to inflict upon me, I would have howled. Standing firm on my two legs, I would have dug out in me the **fundamental complaint** that I felt building up; I would have pushed it up to my throat, up to my mouth from which it would have come out with a dull sound at first like a fog-horn; then it would have swollen like a storm. I would have howled to death and I would never have heard the* *words she was to drop on me like so many* **laming blades.** (my emphasis)

Marie Cardinal has found the words to tell her complaint, to tell it to the world of men, to someone who listens; it is an illustration of the thesis of Jacques Hassoun: 'To be in a position to lodge a complaint, as a privilege granted by men to women, as a privilege that women grant themselves in a society of men.'

The complaint is also at the basis of the analyses of women from which this work originates. These women are pregnant, however, and enjoying because of it a knowledge which is refused to man. But male analysands complain as well; and about what? About not participating in creation, like women, through childbirth. Women want to speak; men want to give birth. Failing which, neurosis or psychosis ensue. One cannot tackle female sexuality without at the same time tackling male sexuality, at the risk of making them into two separate entities.

So woman participates in creation; and it is in that that she is divided, being a creature as well. There lies her share and her suffering; what she receives as her share and what divides her. There also lies the zenith of **jouissance.**

As for man he is both creating and creature, but the dividing line does not go **through** him; it goes **between** the woman and him. Woman is the truth which he questions in order to pierce the secret of creation. (I deliberately retain the typing error: **trouer** instead of **trouver** ['to pierce' instead of 'to find'].)

Woman does not question man. She suffers from being divided and invokes him, as the very ideal of unity. The only thing is that this ideal is what she is not: one. And if she becomes one, she becomes at the same time 'the Other for herself, as she is for him'.

Man is one, through the signifier of his lack, the phallus, which happens to be the symbol of his sexual organ, the penis, which happens to be the organ through which his desire for woman finds a path and is manifested, the instrument which organizes his libido. His **jouissance** is to find the Other in woman and to find as well, even remotely, knowing and having. But this knowledge does not divide him. Man is and remains, as man – and assuming that he exists as a man who would not be a woman as well –, one.

The **jouissance** of woman is the revelation of this one in the Other which makes her one during lovemaking. But to be one, makes her Other, and separates her from her 'mother' in the sense that one says '**la mère du liège**' [lit. 'the mother of the cork'], of the layer between the heart and the bark. Equally, the knowledge given her by the delivery of the child goes through her own and fatal division. Thus, as it was proclaimed to us by Antigone, woman is dedicated to the worship of the Dead; and similarly she offers herself in worship for her fecundity.

No sexual revolution will move these dividing lines, neither that which goes between man and woman, nor that which divides woman. Man will always love that which is put in the place of lack, should it only be a veil. And woman will always love love, which makes Eros one; even if this one should be deceptive. They only touch the truth, one and the other, one through the other, at the risk of losing themselves. To which they ordinarily prefer the affirmation of their respective sufficiency and neurosis.

Man and woman are both born under the regime of lack. However, they are immediately distinguished by the drifting [**dérive** is Lacan's translation of the English 'drive'] that lack of being borrows from having in man, who confines himself to having from the fact that he has a penis. As for woman she confines herself to lack of being; having or not, remaining for her within the register of the imaginary.

Man seeks to fill his lack with a knowledge when the penis is no longer enough; whereas woman, curious and even passionate as she may be, is not wholly consumed, at least with this particular desire. In some way, she already knows about the origin.

Such declarations do not aim to define either a status or an essence. They only state a current opinion, without questioning the perennity of this opinion, even if it means the discovery that this opinion is constant and general.

Man questions the knowledge of woman, a knowledge which is not science, but the omega of science. The sexual knowledge of woman, by the fact of man and on his account, is the beginning of science and of all poetry. We have known that since Dante: man is the scientist; man is the philosopher; man is the poet. Woman is knowledge, 'the other name of God', Lacan might say at this point; 'but then she does not exist', he would add. As for man, his passion for knowledge totalizes him, before totalizing the world. There is in him practically no recognized left over.

'There is no female genius and there can be none . . . woman has no soul . . . women are without both essence and existence; they are not and they are nothing. One is man or woman in as far as one is . . . woman must disappear as woman' (Weininger, 1906).

Indeed. Not a word needs to be removed from this text. But what interests me, if I am an analyst, is why Otto Weininger **wants** to make woman disappear as woman; and why so much passion?

Woman is not, that is agreed; and yet if she disappears, so does the symptom of man as Lacan says. And if there is no longer a symptom, there is no longer a language, and therefore there is no longer a man either.

Thus I could not fail, at the present moment of a reflection that goes through the **champ freudien**, to question myself, as a woman, about the 'what does a woman want?', even if I run the risk of finding out that she, precisely, wants to disappear as woman. A question which does not presuppose that another be resolved, namely: 'What does a man want?'

This is an analytic work, not a philosophical nor a political one. In it we are not very concerned with knowing if woman must make the revolution in order to get the better of a **méconnaissance** [misrecognition, see glossary] which, up to now, may have prevented her from speaking. Neither are we concerned with going over a philosophical discourse which may be erroneous as a result of this misrecognition, and with substituting a better one for it (Irigaray, 1974a).

For a subject in analysis or for an analyst, all discourses are equal; that is to say that no one discourse has any value, except the one in which he has been caught. If the analysis does not cling to the most particular of the desire of the subject – the particular which is defined at every point by his history and told by his symptom – it gets lost in a generalized science

which sterilizes desire. On the other hand it is that which falls into the symptom, from the particularity of the subject, from his most impermeable and ignored abnormality, which is perceptible. As a result of which, suffering generating demand, the analytic work of interpretation and intervention can be done. It is thus from this most particular symptom that the universal of a possible science is introduced; and this is so because of the fact that the symptom affecting the pathological form of suffering already calls upon language and makes the thinking work possible. But there could not be thought from nothing. This constitutes the basis of the cliché according to which the artist is sick and the genius is mad. Indeed they are. They would be; they could have been. Man is thus made that he tells his pain.

My thoughts always merge with what one or another of my analysands say (men **or** women) as well as, through these words, what the analysand that I am says; since one only hears what one is likely to say oneself, but which would remain unsaid without the other.

This telling testifies that it is quite true that woman is caught in male paradigms and systems of representation. But I am not concluding from it that she should not be caught in them. I do not know.

And deliberately, I start listening again: what are they saying, these pregnant women?

Let us posit at first that there is not a specific analysis of children, nor of men or women. Neither is there a specific analysis of pregnant women. There is analysis and an unlimited number of particular analyses. As many analyses as there are analysands. As many symptoms as there are analysands.

1

The blood fable

I call fable that which the subject tells and tells himself. It is
a tale outside the time of the subject's history; but not outside
the time of the analysis, of course, since the fable punctuates
the transference. It is in as far as facts and characters are thus
taken up in a tale and are organized in reference to signifiers
and no longer to a historical truth that they are able to
constitute a fable. It is not even lacking in the apology which
the subject believes he can extract from it, and which comes
down to a discouraged: 'And that's why. . .'

THE FABLE

Anne-Marie, the young woman in analysis whom I shall talk
about here, is twenty-three years old. She is happily married.
She wanted her child; and so did her husband. In order
to have one he even accepted to have some treatment and to
undergo an operation: he had 'haemorrhoids on the testicles'.
As for her she was on the pill – which is not uncommon
nowadays – and had to wait three months before conceiving
the child. That is to say that there was a moment of decision
before the moment of conception; the wish to have a child
was solid.

Anne-Marie became pregnant during the analysis. I was
immediately informed, as I had been informed of the decision.
When the pregnancy was confirmed, she told me at the same
time that she had nothing more to say to me. But it was not
true, as we shall see.

The fable centres around the theme of blood. Not that this
theme gives rise to numerous comments. But it is shown in
biographical facts and dreams of an astonishing precision.
For instance, Anne-Marie suffered from amenorrhoea as well

as constipation, for two years, at the age of eighteen, just like her mother at the same age. I notice, moreover, that her words are scarce and extremely slow. Nothing 'comes out'.

But nothing 'goes in' very easily either, as she is anorectic. I am reminded of the monotonous voice and the hesitant delivery of Blandine some years back, a young girl of twenty, equally anorectic and amenorrhoeic like her mother at the same age.

Anne-Marie's maternal grandfather died of a brain haemorrhage. Anne-Marie's father, a naval officer before becoming a vice-principal in a lycée, also died very suddenly, of a brain haemorrhage: a strange coincidence which immediately suggests to me that there is a displacement upwards in the men on both sides. These vascular accidents lead me to associate Anne-Marie's tale with what a man, also in analysis, told me: 'I was convinced that I had blood clots in the head', he would repeat. He would thus explain the 'terrible migraines' he had around the age of twelve. Of course in girls of that age blood takes another route.

'One year after the death of my father,' Anne-Marie explains, 'I put lipstick on, following a doctor's advice, and my periods came back.' She adds: 'I was engaged.'

This lipstick reminds me of the first dream that Blandine told me: she was playing tennis and she was wearing something red: dress, skirt, jacket. . . A few months later, she announces that she does not dream any longer. She also says that at the time when she used to dream, her dreams were grey, without colour. . . Whereas her mother dreams in colour. . . Yes her mother used to tell her her dreams; and she still tells her when she has her periods. 'You are so lucky,' Blandine replies ('to be able to say that you have your periods' if one is allowed to complete the sentence). In the same way, it is necessary that her mother should know, in return, that she does not eat, does not sleep and does not have her periods. And I must know, me, her analyst, that she does not dream. Periods and dreams can thus be substituted for one another, as an object of refusal, as a no said to the mother.

Equally, Anne-Marie, whose mother 'as usual didn't get it', considers that her mother, warned by her own experience, should have understood. She harbours a tenacious grudge against her. When she appears in her dreams, this mother is always mad or dead. And yet Anne-Marie is the most respectful and docile of the daughters; in addition, she happens to be the eldest daughter of the second marriage; she is perfect and she succeeds in what the eldest daughter of the first marriage does not succeed in; this other eldest has no perfection in any domain. The role of the eldest who succeeds is there of course only for show. It prepares the acting out which will clearly betray its completely external organization or else the liberating enactment [**passage à l'acte**].

With men, 'it's okay'. Anne-Marie married Xavier, a graduate from the Ecole Polytechnique, the son of a general; the army after the navy, therefore, and with a promotion. She imagines him dead when he comes home late. When she was at school, occasionally, she didn't recognize her father coming to collect her, because she had waited for him so much. Her eyes filled with the loved image had probably panicked to the extent of drowning her gaze in the crowd gathered outside. Except for the father there is no other representative of the paternal side of the family in Anne-Marie's account. On the other hand, the maternal side of the family seems inexhaustible: there is the young uncle who terrorized her deliciously, playing with her in the high waves, in spite of her phobia of water, notorious in this family of sailors. She herself states that there is a threat of flood, by water and blood in turn, in her dreams. There is also a sister of the mother, single, and who has attempted to 'take' all her children 'away' from her sister one by one, in order to bring them up in her own way. Anne-Marie became a psychologist and she looks after children. Finally, Anne-Marie's youngest sister, Mirelle, suffers from depression. Anne-Marie is very preoccupied with her, as she reproaches herself for having had, in Mirelle's opinion, a 'privileged status', and thus having maintained her in depression. On the other hand, she makes a link between her sister's mental problem and those that are supposedly threatening her mother. The latter seems so ill that Anne-Marie is afraid, as she will say much later, of leaving her children with her mother. (She will have two daughters during her analysis.)

When she announces her first pregnancy, her discourse changes totally. It is the analysis now which causes anxiety: 'Am I analysable? I don't have any more dreams.' (Surprising denial, for she dreams a lot, as we shall see later.) 'What am I doing here? Am I pregnant?' It is thus in the shape of a question that she told me the news. Presented in that way, the pregnancy seems to me very much like a resistance.

Shortly before her pregnancy, she dreamt that she begot (instead of 'stepped over') a dangerous foot bridge ['**engendrait**' instead of '**enjambait**']. And shortly thereafter, she dreams that she gives birth prematurely to a girl, whereas she is expecting a boy. There is a very blue sea nearby. Threatening, invading sea. Her eldest brother says: 'We must close the window. There is a risk of the baby drowning.' Then the baby is dipped in a bathtub; 'it's very frightening'. One would wonder why so much fear, if it wasn't a dream.

So, she dreams; some time later, she also has a clearly homosexual dream. It is not the first one. She is nevertheless very surprised about it. I don't understand, she says (like her mother who did not understand, probably!). The dream is as clear as it is short: 'I have erotic feelings with a little girl.' At the end of the month, she has another dream which she calls 'horrible': a little girl on a bicycle; there is a mountain race; she falls; at first there is nothing, then suddenly blood spurts out everywhere very heavily; she is covered in blood.

Amenorrhoea can be seen as a reaction of fright: fear of running blood, of flood, of the terrible sea, of the overwhelming wave, etc.

The husband is a bit forgotten, she does not feel very much like making love. Sexual intercourse is becoming less frequent. He works too much; then, he gets on her nerves. Finally he is too small. She dreamt one day that 'he was smaller than the norm' and that she was going to have abormal children. She feels attracted to other men. She, who is so moralistic and even bourgeois, starts dreaming, without really admitting it, of communal life. There is a young man she fancies, a friend of the couple. She remembers also that there was another man around, when she met Xavier. Pregnancy turns her into a kind of universal woman; a woman for everyone, at a pinch.

Finally she once again has a dream which recalls the first

anxiety dreams: a car which immediately follows theirs is
swallowed up by a huge wave; the sea is threatening; there is
a dangerous **bridge** which must be crossed in order to reach
the family home, which is on the lake. This summer she had a
terrible anxiety attack because her husband had gone fishing
at sea: 'I was in a real panic,' she says. When the baby is not
moving, she is afraid that he is dead. He has to move all the
time.

A new theme appears: the theme of the gift. 'We used to give
my mother gifts, she hardly responded.'

Although she doesn't quite express it, these dreams say
in her place that she fears labour like a ground swell, like
a rushing wave of blood. During the two years in which her
periods had stopped, Anne-Marie got rid of the very sign of
femaleness (whereas the most obvious symptom of Marie Cardinal is the continuous flow of blood, without intervals). It is
because, for Anne-Marie, woman is guilty. **Her mother stole
her father away from a dead woman.** She married a widower,
who moreover had lost a son from that first marriage. Not
having a child is being punished, Anne-Marie tells me. But as
soon as she expects to have one, she panics. Death threatens.
Anne-Marie **oscillates between not being a woman or dying a
bloody death because woman is guilty of theft and murder**.
The gifts that she gives her mother in her dreams seem very
much like propitiatory gifts offered to an awesome goddess.

The return to the mother brings us back to something quite
archaic. Anne-Marie came to analysis to escape from her
mother: I am here; she has nothing to fear; at least she believes
so, in spite of her dreams. When she is pregnant her mother
is not the first person she tells. And yet her mother brought
her a child shortly before her own pregnancy: and precisely in
the shape of a short delusion; she thought she was pregnant,
when she had not made love. Anne-Marie was very shaken
by this premonitory happening. But then 'all that's over;
I'm the one who's pregnant, not my mother; and it's not my
mother's child, although she asked to look after the child after
the birth, to help me. But I won't leave it with her. Anyway,
I would be much too afraid.' 'Afraid of what?' I asked. 'She
forgets things, she is not well; I would fear for the child.'

As for Xavier, he is very happy; he takes care of everything. He dreams of the baby every night. It must be added to what was said above that Anne-Marie, for her part, dreams that she sleeps her pregnancy to its term; to wake up, in one of her dreams, would be to give birth. But in the dreamt awakening, the baby is still not there. Anxiety. Then she wakes up, and upon waking up for real, she realizes that she is pregnant and that the child is still in her belly.

She used me and she used analysis in order to evade the problem. I am in some way the Holy Ghost and Xavier is Joseph. As for her, I will not say that she is the Virgin Mary, because, in truth, she feels she never was a virgin, she never had to be deflowered. But above all the 'I'm no longer afraid' testifies to a permanent state of denial: she wants to sleep. Through me, it is with her father that, as the eldest daughter, sure of her prerogatives (she is 'privileged') and at the expense of her 'mad' but omnipotent mother, she has made the child.

PREGNANCY

After this account of the fable which I kept as brief as possible, I shall examine a few points which seem to me worth thinking about:

1. The conception of the child constitutes here an acting out during the treatment. The child is used like a plug to close the question: If I don't have my periods, am I still a woman? It is also a way of placing the analyst with her back to the wall: are you going to intervene or not?

2. When a woman becomes pregnant during analysis, it can be said that the child is in imagination the analyst's child. 'Analyst's child', it is a manner of speaking, as one says 'the Oedipal child', with the understanding that the Oedipus is not Oedipus and cannot really have a child. The analyst can do it all; but it is not as a real begetter that he is a parent here. Besides it happens that I am a woman. Were the analyst a man, the analytic problematic would be in no way different.

3. There is an homosexual crisis and a return to the mother.

4. The fantasized child is the penis stolen from the progenitor.

5. There is change of sex between the spouses, and I play on the word 'change' [change] in order not to say 'a changing' [changement] which would imply a real modification (which

is obviously not in question, even though it may seem like it, as
echoed in *Les mamelles de Tirésias* [*The Breasts of Tiresias*]
(Apollinaire, 1946)). I say 'change' in order not to say, either,
'sexual exchange' [**échange sexuel**], but in order to evoke
the expression '**donner le change**' [as a hunting metaphor:
'to throw someone off the scent'; thus here: 'to confuse signs
of identity']. This sex change [**change de sexe**] turns the
woman into a father-mother, she becomes masculine. As
for the man, he becomes maternal and feminine. There is,
for each, identification with the sex of the other in order to
compensate for the failure of the exchange.

6. All these events result in a strong resistance to the analysis.

These six points are going to order the following reflections.

Resistance and passage à l'acte (points 6 and 1)

I shall begin with the first and last points together because
resistance to the analysis is what this young woman and
others expressed clearly at first, as soon as they knew they
were pregnant. '**I have nothing more to say . . . everything
is okay . . . I feel like stopping the analysis . . . and I would
gladly leave you with a slap in the face** . . . (at the age of
sixteen, Anne-Marie slapped her mother; after which she left
home). . . . **I am afraid to go on talking . . . pregnancy is a
private affair . . .**' Such is the substance of what I was given
to hear. But, naturally, analysis went on and dreams would
contradict what was deliberately being said. 'I cannot stop
dreaming of you', says one. Another wants me to be 'witness'
to the birth of the child. Some are sorry to go on holiday
because, when the child moves, I will not be there and they will
not be able to let me know. I am the one who is first informed
of the pregnancy, after the husband, but before the mother.
Even the one who fears that she might be having a phantom
pregnancy lets me know that her periods have stopped, all
the while fearing that she might have to admit to a disappointment. Anne-Marie dreams that I grab her; I have a bottle of
red liquid in my hand; I am persecuting her.

Another one states more specifically: 'I had already fantasized quite a bit about the person I saw in the entrance.
I thought it was your daughter; then I saw your grandchild
and as it happens we conceived the child right afterwards.'

Another one says: 'You have been present from the start of the analysis. I have done everything in the analysis: my un-marriage, the child, my next marriage. . . You are someone who contains me and whom I contain. It is merged. It reminds me a bit of a mirror, but it has a volume.'

The contradiction between the liveliness of the transfer-ence and the expressed wish to put an end to the analysis is only on the surface. If analysis actually stops, it is necessary that the bond with the analyst be in some way preserved in the real. What better way than by turning the analyst into the spiritual parent? Hence the form assumed by the transference.

Return to the mother (point 3)

In this transference phenomenon I am, as the analyst, con-fused with the character of the mother (at first).

From the beginning of the pregnancy I hear words such as these: 'I think about my mother non-stop. What could her love life have been?' One had a phantom pregnancy like her mother: 'And I was only born six years later' she adds, as if she was already there during the phantom pregnancy. The other one (Anne-Marie) was amenorrhoeic for two years like her mother.

She has a dream at the beginning of her pregnancy (men-tioned above) in which she 'experiences erotic feelings with a little girl' – a dream in which it is possible to locate the return of the excitement of the little girl with her own mother – she does not understand; she has never been homosexual; she never thought of it. Another one says: 'I don't want to get married for the sake of it. I want to be a married mother for my mother.' We must hear this 'for'; because, according to the daughter, the mother is frigid; she is therefore a married mother and not a wife. Anne-Marie cannot think of her par-ents as a couple. Another one, a homosexual, dreams right away that she is having a shit (these are her words and she insists on them) with her mother-in-law when her husband arrives: everyone is happy.

I kept the following memory for the end. It was recollected in the second month of Anne-Marie's pregnancy, while she was announcing her remarriage and the change of name that would result (for she too, like her mother, had two husbands; but she got a divorce the first time).

A very violent memory is coming back to me . . . I had cheated at school; I was six. The teacher made me copy out: **I shall not cheat** *. . . I signed the copy with my mother's name. What a fuss . . . Another thing: I was sleeping in a renovated attic. One day, on the door which led to the landing where my bedroom was, I saw my mother's name written in pencil. I told her. She said: 'I don't understand'; but I'm sure it was true.*

There is moreover a whole story around Anne-Marie's maiden name and my name.

Return to the mother, homosexuality and transference are thus strongly articulated.

The stolen penis and the sex change [changement de sexe] (points 4 and 5)
The events I have just mentioned bring about a certain distancing from the husband . . . 'I was frigid just after I thought I was pregnant', Anne-Marie states, she who, up to then, had been very tender towards her husband; and she admits that he gets on her nerves; then he works too much, and then he is too small. The father worked too much; he was always away and he was small. Another one says: 'In relation to my husband, I am now very withdrawn.' Yet another one dreams that she sucks the genitals of a homosexual and that she is left with 'a piece of chicken skin or something similar' in her mouth; she also speaks of a goose neck, then of testicles and foetus. Another one speaks of the first man she loved and she states that she will never again feel such excitement: and of course she does not mean the husband!

Soon I hear of a husband who would like to turn into a midwife; who dreams of the baby every night and would like to carry it; he attends all the prenatal classes; he even says that he would like to 'switch with his wife' [changer avec sa femme]. A man, in a psychodrama group, mimes his wife's termination on medical grounds; he says that he cannot get over it; he cannot want any more children; it is as if he had aborted himself; he becomes heavily depressed. (For every-

thing concerning paternity and the 'psychoses of paternity'
see Ebtinger and Renoux, 1967.)

'It's amazing how much I dream of the phallus out of its
"proper" place,' says a young woman shortly before giving
birth (she is using phallus for penis). And another one: 'My
mother offered me a penis which wasn't attached to a body;
flying penis and testicles.' It is a dream that the analysand
said she had forgotten.

What all these texts say in the end is that the husband is
forsaken; that he feels himself turning into a woman; that the
woman is now self-sufficient. That the penis which has been
stolen from the father by the frigid mother is now given to the
daughter at the expense of the husband. This may seem a bit
contrived because I am obliged to condense a lot and drop
many other texts. But what follows will, I believe, throw some
light on this beginning.

A NEW READING

If the child is the analyst's child, there must have been a **fec-
und moment** when it was conceived. At that time the analyst
must have let something happen or take place, if only by her
silence; I looked through my notes, in search of the fecund
moment.

In fact, in Anne-Marie's case, I was absent at the time of
conception. Absent also at the time of the decision which was
made three months earlier. The conception took place in the
country, away from Paris, during a short holiday. As for the
decision, it is all the more loaded with meaning as it had to
be kept for three months, at the end of which the child was
conceived.

Moreover, something important happened for Anne-Marie
in the month which preceded the decision and the two months
that followed: the couple had a beautiful woman friend stay
with them. A **ménage à trois** was immediately set up: at the
start the friend preferred the woman of the couple (Anne-
Marie) who, herself, said she was attracted to her. At first,
the friend expressly refused to make love with the husband,
stating that, all in all, she would prefer Anne-Marie. But
Anne-Marie didn't make up her mind and what had to happen
happened. So the friend and the husband make love in the

marital bed and Anne-Marie, lying next to them, falls asleep. It was clear that he had to 'sow his wild oats', she says of Xavier. Which would mean that she did not think of him quite as a man yet.

Listening to her, I recall that she once had a dream very similar in situation. 'She was in bed with her father and mother who could not make love; and she put her hands between her mother's thighs. Her father then faded away.' When telling this dream, she added: 'They should have got a divorce before I was born', then, in the same session: 'I don't understand how two and two make four'; then 'the couple was between my mother and me'. Who then was **between** the couple she would have liked to form with her friend?

In another dream of the same series, she was teaching a young boy of fourteen – who is in therapy with her – how to make love. She was holding him in her arms, on her lap.

If we return to the threesome, there were two possible solutions. The first one, which could have been expected, was that a homosexual couple was constituted next to an obliging husband. The second was that a **ménage à trois** was organized in which the husband would make love with the friend in front of his wife. It was no doubt what the husband was hoping for. But Anne-Marie fell asleep. In fact she wanted to help her husband, towards whom she behaves in a maternal way, as she does with her young patient. Besides, she describes her husband as a boyish looking man. Her first husband was also smaller than she; he was ill and even took drugs.

When she is not maternal, Anne-Marie becomes a man: I am a man with women, she says, and a woman with men. It is a manner of speaking. Her only opportunity to feel like a woman would be with men who are black, tall and bearded (she knows quite a few of them, and is still attracted to them), but then nothing happens because she feels like a little girl. The result of all of this is that between **little girl** and **mother/father**, there is **no room for the woman**. Hence, Anne-Marie telling me also that she did not have a 'developer [**révélateur**] to speak of her father': these are her own words; one may think that I have not been this woman, this developer.

I have not provided her with this particular signifier. Up to then, she told me around the same time, I considered you as a vice-principal (one recalls that her father is vice-principal in a lycée), then it changed. Indeed, the analyst has become the mother 'that one makes dead', if one does 'terrible' things. 'Rightly or wrongly,' she says, 'I have the feeling that you wouldn't agree if I took drugs or if I joined a sexually liberated commune. And that would make my mother dead and you too. And that I cannot do.'

So I end up having chosen with her the so-called normal path and having averted the 'terrible' choices. I also met her homosexual transference with a refusal. Occasionally, she reminds me that I have never called her by her first name, which she would have liked very much; but she doesn't regret that I was distant, and she now expresses satisfaction that I was. The turning point was obviously the affair with the friend as a third party. **No longer knowing — as a good hysteric — if she was a man or a woman, she chose to force herself to be a woman by making a child.** Thus, she thought, the issue was settled. The father was obviously a man, and Anne-Marie obviously a woman. That is what I call '**donner le change**' ['throwing off the scent'].

She had also spoken about 'provoking things in order to understand' and 'putting her back to the wall'. All of this betrays acting out.

To sum up: Anne-Marie decided to have a child in order to avoid declaring herself homosexual and in order to make herself become a woman without recourse to a man. I mean to say that it is not the sexual encounter which decided the sex, nor did it confirm it; and yet, that is what she would have needed, since she experiences herself as 'not quite a woman'. There is something which did not happen and which no doubt would have been the revelation of her femininity. And she says: 'I don't have a developer to speak of the father.' She absolutely does not know that what she lacks is to be able to speak of the woman, as a woman, so much the lack is lack. At least that is what I am putting forward, and it may be problematic.

In any case, before she was pregnant, the delivery was fantasized with terror as a haemorrhage. I don't think one can say that she feared it and hoped for it as the deflowering

which hadn't occurred at the time, since she stated never
having been a virgin – although, why not? – but rather as the
expulsion of something she had in her and which would empty
her as it came out. I put forward the hypothesis, given the
context, that it was the penis: the penis against the emptiness,
a plug to prevent the body from emptying.

During the preliminary interviews, she had told me that she
was looking after children and wanted to become an analyst.
She had even asked for reassurance, which, of course, I had
not given her. I should have done more, and analysed at the
time a parallel which became obvious later on, namely:
— wanting to speak and not being able to,
— wanting to write and not being able to,
— wanting to be an analyst and not being able to,
because the analyst does not want it; because the mother does
not want it. And I translate now:
— wanting to be a woman and not being able to.

I probably do not allow her either. I do not make it possible;
and what I do not give her, she takes by force, by making a
child which she brings me. She also says that I have blocked
her. I therefore cornered her into acting out. Moreover, she
imagined that if she revealed herself mad, I would not let her
become an analyst. Curious outcome for an analysis which
had begun under the theme of health. What mattered for
Anne-Marie was to become an analyst, her symptoms being
brought forward, patently, only to support her demand.

If the child has been conceived away from me, it is no doubt
in order to present me with a **fait accompli**. But there is
nothing irretrievable, under the circumstances. The analysis
continues.

A PARADIGM

So she made a child because she didn't know how to be a woman otherwise; and she made it at the time when she had other
choices: homosexuality and the excesses of the commune on
the one hand; on the other hand, the order that I represented:
order, and not woman.

Besides, the child was not only wanted, but programmed;
during these three months of enforced waiting, we had all
the time to start up another discourse. But no, the child is

conceived; then it is announced and offered to me. I become confused with the recovered mother. The husband becomes feminine. As for her, she becomes a mother, not a woman. The child will be the false guarantee of the respective sex of each and the symbol of their union.

Thus it blocks the access to the symbolic, since such access can only be achieved, precisely, through the encounter with the other, of which the other sex is a modality. We recognize here something that the psychoanalyst Eliane Amado Levy-Valensi says: namely that the man in the Christian couple is castrated; the woman is magnified as mother; the child is regarded as sacred and as a symbol, at the expense of the couple. The woman, thus, gives herself the penis under the guise of the child without having to assert her demand for the penis as such. She is the one who brings about the union, to her benefit, through a kind of misappropriation.

For me it is not a question of unmaking the child after having allowed it to be made. Besides, after a period of some time when the analysand was happily floating on her back on the couch, the work started again and now it doesn't seem hampered by the other work, of the pregnancy. From time to time the analysand falls asleep again, in line with the dream mentioned earlier. She is delighted she no longer has her major symptom, death anxiety. The child has worked well as a plug. But the euphoria (which reminded me of Faulkner's pregnant woman in *Light in August* (1932)) does not last. Disquiet and analysis start up again. Anne-Marie reflects. She goes back with me over the time of the decision and the conception to see what did happen there.

As a conclusion, I propose the fictitious genealogical line which follows:

Mother: immortal and omnipotent goddess, mad.

Father: not mad, but sick, afflicted, threatened with death.

Their analysand daughter: looks after children – usurpation.

The husband: small and thin or young or sexually handicapped.

The other man: powerful and bearded, whom the analysand never meets, for the good reason that she is afraid of him.

The analyst: woman (or/and man).

Their child: whose child?

This line has the value of a paradigm, although all pregnant women do not have a mad mother, a sick father and a small husband in the proper sense of those terms. But in some way, one can say that they are indeed mad, sick, bearded and small. All little girls in primary school sing a very significant song to this effect:

My mother gave me a husband
My God what a man, what a small man!
My mother gave me a husband
My God what a man, how small he is!

The husband is thus in some way small, he is not a big man; the paradigm is only apparently exaggerated. No doubt the attributes could be differently distributed: but then the whole set would shift. In any case, the child remains the last stake. Can anyone speak more harshly than Goethe of the child who is, nevertheless, legitimate and conceived in love? Let us recall what he says in *Elective Affinities* (1809): 'Let me throw a veil,' he says to his new love, Odile, 'over this fatal hour which gave being to this child. . . Why would those harsh words not be uttered: this child is the fruit of a double adultery. . .' Indeed, they were four when it was conceived and no longer two. One knows the story of the four partners of *Elective Affinities* and the chemical laws regulating their swaps: if one brings together A and B and another couple just as close, C and D, there fatally occurs a **chassé-croisé** such that A is joined to C; and B to D. If the birth of a child should follow, whose child is it?

Edward, Charlotte's husband, is neither sick nor small, but he is already middle-aged and the marriage was not a love match. The Captain, since that's what he is, is necessarily the 'bearded' and powerful lover. The young Odile stands in rather well for the beautiful friend of the Anne-Marie–Xavier couple. And the Captain is Edward's friend, just as one of the powerful men (analyst or lover) who subjugates Anne-Marie, has been and remains the friend and the ideal of her husband.

The child that Charlotte brings into the world, after she and her husband have renounced their passion for the Captain and Odile respectively (but couldn't one speak as well of

Charlotte's love for Odile and Edward's for the Captain?) looks like both Odile and the Captain. 'It is the fruit of a double moral adultery', writes Jeanne Ancelet-Hustache (1976), after Goethe.

The epilogue is tragic: Odile drops the child in the lake and starves herself to death. Edward commits suicide.

In analysis, the so-called child of the analyst is only the fruit of the transference, not of a moral incest; provided at least that the analyst was able to indicate in the transference that his own desire was not a desire for a child: it is on this condition that the child will be free of any transferential alienation.

2
Pregnancy and femininity

FROM this case a theoretical work can be initiated around the following points:

1. Pregnancy as a narcissistic crisis (object relation during pregnancy and after);

2. The taking apart, during pregnancy, of the specular image manufactured at the mirror stage, and its various outcomes;

3. The symbolic outcome: from two to three;

4. The sex change in order to compensate for the failure of the exchange and the impossibility of sexual relation;

5. And yet, woman speaks (commentary on a schema of Lacan's);

6. In brief, she goes from imaginary division to symbolic castration. How?

PREGNANCY AS A NARCISSISTIC CRISIS

Pregnancy and delivery, like coitus and defecation, are fundamentally animal phenomena. Freud says it, insistently (1912): 'The excremental is all too intimately and inseparably bound up with the sexual.' And also: 'The genitals themselves have not taken part in the development of the human body in the direction of beauty. . .' Which is another way of putting it, and a way of saying something more. 'They have remained animal', Freud adds; and also 'love has remained in essence just as animal as it ever was'.

Pregnancy as well. If 'the animal is in the world like water in water' according to the wonderful formulation of Georges Bataille, where then does the cut from animal to man occur? Where does the separation take place? What about man and woman in the world? It is an issue we will have to take up later (cf. the 'separation', below, p.70). There is no point in wondering if woman is more animal than man. For women like Madame Bovary, man is a beast; and there is the tale of *Beauty and the Beast*. But a lot of men have a horror of women: of the female.

And yet both sexes collude in magnifying a group of phenomena: coitus, pregnancy and delivery gathered under the name of childbirth. They have even made religions out of them. Whereas there is no question of magnifying defecation, except in making the product unrecognizable as gold and money; and even so Freud was needed for the equation: faeces = money = penis to be established. Orality receives some fine transpositions; defecation lends itself only to perverse exploitation. In contrast, childbirth is forced into the register of the sublime. One cannot bear animality in relation to mother and child. Abortion, whether induced or not, is probably the rejection of this something not yet sexed or named; rejection in other words, of an unnamable, of a non symbolizable.

The way woman has always been concerned with her beauty – which, according to Gide in *Corydon* (1920), goes against the natural laws of the male being more ornate than the female – is certainly a fierce denial of her animality. Modesty is another form of that denial, a mask . . . (see chapter 6).

Certainly women do not admit easily to their animality.

The **Précieuses** [characters from Molière's play, *Les Précieuses ridicules*] didn't like naturalness, nor – already! – did the wives of the first Christians of whom St Jerome says 'they speak between their teeth or with the edge of their lips, whispering and only half pronouncing words, because they consider all that is natural to be crude'. 'These women,' he goes on, 'even corrupt language' ('Letter to Eustochium', quoted by Havelock Ellis in *Sex and Marriage*, 1951). They do not want to call a spade a spade. They do not want to name. Nomenclature is a fact of men. Language does not have this divine function for women; and that wouldn't matter, even if it became corrupted, if it was not for the fact that they end up using it for all kinds of purposes (including camouflage) in the same way as make up, finery, trinkets and other masks necessary to the female economy.

Now, put to the test of pregnancy, beauty as an idol shatters.

What happens then for woman? Can she bear to see what was hidden under the mask?

Freud provides the answer in his analysis of narcissism (1914) although there is no mention of the pregnant woman in it. During pregnancy, a woman goes through a narcissistic crisis, accompanied by all the dangers of regression and imbalance that narcissism implies. One observes, through the sequence of pregnancy and delivery, the same phases that Freud pointed out, namely:

1. A withdrawal of libido (previously directed towards the husband) and a flowing back of this libido towards the imaginary ego;

2. A paranoid delusion of grandeur, woman experiencing herself as the creator;

3. A coming down of the delusion after delivery, brought about by a stasis of the libido, itself following up on the failure of the delusion. Depression sets in in the place of the delusion;

4. Another delusion, mixed with a wish for murder, may then break out as an alternative to depression. There is refusal of the real child. ('Real' is used here on the one hand as it is in everyday language, where it is opposed to the imaginary, and on the other hand, as a reference to Freud for whom it is opposed as object to the narcissistic object. Its use is thus conventional and not philosophical.)

Freud (1914) speaks of an 'internal working over of libido which has returned to the ego' adding that 'perhaps it is only when the megalomania fails that the damming-up of libido in the ego becomes pathogenic'.

Indeed, the pregnant woman is not ill, except for some cases of neuroses with which I am not especially concerned here. She is even unusually blooming, particularly during the last months when the child moves; for it becomes then a perfect alibi: it keeps on feeding the delusion of the mother, as a part of herself which came to complement her imaginary ego, and it is already real, since it moves.

In brief, however real, however alive, it nevertheless goes on functioning as an imaginary object which has come to fulfil a very old desire. It functions literally as a plug and cancels out anxiety. The woman is full; she is even full to 'bursting' point. Fantasies of bursting come then to upset this nice balance. But it is only at the time of birth – when the real child takes up in the outside the place it occupied inside – that the gap between the imaginary object and the real object opens up its disturbing hiatus. Not that the child is better or worse than the dream child. Not even that it is a boy or a girl or the other way round; it is only of another register: it is real.

This particular real, which can no longer be assimilated, is given properly speaking as a monster: as a separate thing showing itself to be frightening in its otherness and its aggressivity, whereas it was still 'immanent' to the mother not long ago; we are borrowing this word from Georges Bataille (1973): not that it belongs to him exclusively; but Georges Bataille gives it a scope which interests us here: 'In the end,' he writes, 'we perceive each appearance – subject (ourselves), animal, spirit, world – at once from inside and from outside, both as a continuity in relation to ourselves and as object'. The child is this object par excellence which is no longer either inside or outside and which turns the mother into an outside, an object for herself. Separation has occurred and immanence is done away with; the child is no longer like water in water. It is well and truly **brought into the world**, in the world, and from there it so much threatens the balance of the new mother that it triggers, at best, some slight depression, and at worst postnatal psychoses mixed with murderous wishes.

Let us take up Freud's analysis again (1914); according to him, woman is essentially narcissistic and little inclined to object love: 'Strictly speaking, it is only themselves that such women love with . . . intensity.' She is particularly self-sufficient when she is pregnant. Some women only feel good when pregnant. Freud, however, acknowledges that for woman, the child is a real object.

A human being has originally two sexual objects – himself and the woman who nurses him. . . Even for narcissistic women, whose attitude towards men remains cool, there is a road which leads to complete object-love. In the child which they bear, a part of their own body confronts them like an extraneous object, to which, starting out from their narcissism, they can then give complete object-love.

It remains true, however, that the child, inasmuch as it is

imaginarily given by a daughter to her mother, cannot constitute this full object-love. A failure of objectification which is one
of the causes of abortion. And as, at one time or another, the
child remains the unnamable, there is no pregnant woman
who completely escapes the threat of abortion. When is the
foetus recognized as a child by the pregnant woman? Hence,
no doubt, Freud's severity in respect of parental love which
one would wish sublime and which he qualifies as childish,
even if he acknowledges, let us repeat, that the child opens up
for women a possible access to the real.

They have another access to the real, when the wish for a
penis 'changes into the wish for a **man**, and thus puts up with
the man as an appendage to the penis' (Freud, 1917). (Man
as appendage to the penis! Feminists would not put it any
other way.) For all that, this double pathway is double only in
theory, because there is equivalence and possible substitution
between the three terms: faeces, penis and child. 'In the wish
for a baby, an anal-erotic and a genital impulse ("envy for a
penis") converge' (Freud, 1917).

The myth of the narcissistic adventure of pregnancy was
found by Hoffmansthal in *Die Frau ohne Schatten* ['the
woman without a shadow']. *Die Frau ohne Schatten* (1919)
is contemporary with the mature works of Freud. This **ohne
Schatten** reminded me of the word **schattenhaft** (shadowy),
chosen, as it happens, by Freud to describe what is unanalys-
able in woman. 'Everything in the sphere of this first at-
tachment to the mother seemed to me so difficult to grasp in
analysis – so grey with age and shadowy and almost impossible
to revivify – that it was as if it had succumbed to an especially
inexorable repression' (Freud, 1931). Now, it seems that it is
this bond that woman cannot let go of.

What is this 'woman without a shadow'? A woman who cannot have a child because she has no shadow. She is the wife of
a handsome emperor who spends his time hunting: it is thus,
as ever hunting, that catching her he caught his first prey: the
daughter of the invisible and immortal god Keikobad.

But this god loved a simple mortal woman, just for as long as
it took for him to become a father: she does not appear in the
story at all and, through not appearing, she leaves a 'blank'
which is the very place around which the drama revolves.

The empress, daughter of the god, is thus also the daughter of a human mother, who passed on to her this desire of giving birth which is impossible to satisfy. It would no doubt have been necessary for this maternal bond to remain alive for the empress to be able to have a child. But instead of her earthly mother all she has is a nurse of darkness.

The meaning of the disparity between the parental couple can already be glimpsed: omnipresent father, absent mother: in order to give birth, a woman must be the daughter of an earthly mother and not only of a father-god. If she wants to give birth at all cost – if one wants to give birth at all cost – she is forced to go and rob the shadow of an earthly woman, the shadow of her mother, outside the celestial dwelling of her father. At any rate, this is how I interpret the myth through what has been transmitted to us by Hoffmansthal.

It is only on earth, amongst humans, that the empress may replace this lost shadow, memory of the 'dark continent' as Freud might say; which is why the services of the nurse are indispensable. She takes on the dark design of providing it for the empress; dark, because it is a matter of offering to a mortal a fraudulent exchange; the shadow for the finery, the shadow being the precious goods; and the finery pure illusion. The nurse, tool of the empress, like Oenone for Phedra, takes the responsibility on herself, out of love for this daughter for whom she has been a kind of mother through the eclipse of another woman.

There are thus three levels in Hoffmansthal's world, as in Giraudoux's whose divine characters are equally fond of coming back to earth. But this threefold division is probably true of any mythical universe where the three levels are present: that of the god, Keikobad; that of the heroes, the emperor and empress; and that of the humans: the dyer Barak and his wife. What strikes me in Giraudoux as in Hoffmansthal is that these three levels reproduce quite well the imaginary family diagram which I laid out earlier, and according to which the woman is pregnant from at least three males:

1. A god, great ancestor or family hero;
2. A husband, small, nice and castrated;
3. A black lover, powerful and bearded = the Beast.

All these adjectives are obviously purely 'moral' in spite of their seeming physical precision. One only needs to see what determines choice in psychodramas to be convinced – the choice always being so disconcerting, because of the gap between the description made of the spouse and the person chosen to take their place.

Through this game of the threefold begetter woman repays man in kind, man who, as Lacan says, takes all the women one by one, in an attempt to have **the Woman** (and none of them is). (There is a fourth one – when the woman is in analysis – who is liable to be one or the other of the three males, as well as the analysand's mother on top of it: that is the psychoanalyst. This is why we have put forward the view that the child of the pregnant woman in analysis is always the analyst's child. As for Freud, he states that the husband always has second place in a woman's heart, after the father. Thus she goes looking for a complement outside of her husband.)

To return to Hoffmansthal's myth, his empress has much too pure a heart to go along with the exchange plotted by the nurse. By refusing the bargain she goes against another evil will: that of her father, the immortal god, who uses the nurse, even if it means leaving her to perish, should she fail. Keikobad himself wants his daughter to give birth, indeed. It is not for nothing that he once went to find a mortal. This myth is the opposite of that of Prometheus or of Icarus: it is not man who wants to steal the divine fire, or simply to fly [voler: both 'to steal' and 'to fly'], it is God who wants to steal a mortal shadow. It is the empress, his daughter, who wants to descend, to fall (pregnant), to put on weight, to acquire substance. In any case, Keikobad will punish the couple, if his daughter does not give birth, by turning her hunter husband into stone (then weight will really win out!). Indeed this childbirth story cannot end. No childbirth can be conceived of, if it is not inscribed in an infinite chain of childbirths. If his daughter doesn't have a child, it is in vain that he, the god, has a daughter: he returns to his immortal god's nothingness.

As for the tale, it has an end. Barak's wife, not satisfied with adorning herself with cheap jewels which repay her for her treason, attempts to seduce a fake prince, and Barak catches her in the act. His manly honour at stake, he changes into a superb and generous lion and brandishes his sword against his wife. It seems that, suddenly, she has the revelation of the "'real' penis of her husband, displayed at last in the symbol. She falls on her knees in front of him and begs for his forgiveness.

The empress seeing the shadow escaping her (shadow that she was loath to grab through bartering) renounces it completely and is only concerned with freeing her jailed husband. She goes back to the high estate to implore her father. Keikobad remains inflexible and with good reason: if his daughter is childless, he will never have any descendants. Even more inflexible than he (like father, like daughter), she pronounces a 'I do not want' which robs the terrible father of his power. The husband comes back to life at that very moment: he moves. And the empress miraculously throws a shadow. The chorus of the children to be born can then be heard.

The conclusion of the story — both moral and romantic — is easy to draw: love is stronger than death. But the meaning of the myth is elsewhere. It tells us that only the woman who has a shadow can give birth; and if her own mother has disappeared (as the human mother of the empress has) and cannot therefore pass this shadow on to her, she still has the possibility of stealing one; this solution, however, has regrettable consequences and all that is left for the woman who wants to give birth is symbolically to kill her father-god while acknowledging the limited and only human manliness of her husband. (Otto Rank (1932) gives a completely different interpretation of this tale.)

This myth also tells us that the woman cannot give her child the sole **name** of its own father, and that the desire of the father (that his daughter should have a child) is not enough to make her fertile. The daughter must say no to the father. As for stealing a shadow, that is not possible, although there are shadows to spare amongst women 'besotted with their own bodies'. All that is left for the woman then is to say: yes to a man, after having said no to her father; and this could be translated in different terms. . .

But still: what is this shadow? To take things literally, it is the shadow of the body, its darkness. It is thick and heavy; it doesn't let light through. And the body of the woman doesn't either, no doubt. The body is equally dense or equally empty.

But for man, the issue is not to become two or to divide into two; and if the human body is a sack, to see to it that it is no longer empty. The play of empty and full is, on the contrary, at the core of the female imaginary. Woman has a good method for filling up the emptiness: to become fat or to become pregnant. 'Iω heavy',* such is the humorous title that a writer gave a tale written in honour of his pregnant wife.

Heavy, this is how the Giraffe (of whom I shall speak again) wants to be. Heavy hiking shoes could weigh her down, at a pinch. . . This displacement would be humorous if humour could be involuntary. It exonerates the Giraffe (conveniently) from facing pregnancy and from demanding that the husband, who for the time being is sterile, should seek treatment. Who would think that such a trick would work?

It doesn't completely work and the Giraffe is not altogether sure that she is not responsible for the sterility of the couple. Now, if she had a child, she would become a woman. She has reached a stalemate. Especially as she cannot become fat, since she is anorectic, as Binswanger's Ellen West (1944) who said: 'Something in me is revolted at the thought of becoming fat.' Which Binswanger interpreted as the fear of becoming pregnant. Eating, becoming fat, being made pregnant; feeding, being fed are the terms of a completely transitivist oral drive.

If the husband is cured one day and thus summons her to prove her femininity, the Giraffe will feel 'cornered'. But he doesn't get better, and he even becomes fat and gives her the feeling that he is becoming feminine. 'I have the feeling that I touch my mother,' she says. The Giraffe is similar both to the Bovary-like wife of Barak and to the empress. She would like to weigh more, but without putting on weight; to be a star, but also a mother.

When she no longer speaks of weight, she speaks of measure. She doesn't want to have a child, she says, so as not to 'run the risk of gaining a couple of inches around the waist'. It is clear that with these additional inches she would lose

---

* 'Iω' was the name of a goddess and 'Iω heavy' is a witticism; cf. 'eau lourde', that is to say 'oil', where eau sounds like io. A pregnant woman in fact is heavy.

herself as identical to herself. She cannot bear the thought
of seeing her image altering, becoming other. She would no
longer recognize herself in it and would therefore cease to be.
The Giraffe, like all women who aspire to be leading ladies or
stars (it is the radiating image of the empress) has the dream
of becoming an indestructible shape and of killing the beas
dream of narcissistic beauty.

But the image is inconsistent; there is nothing inside. It is
the luminous double in opposition to the shadow; the glorious
body of the empress before conception. Once the specular
image is broken, and beyond it, it is possible for the daughter
to find the obscure double, the body of the mother; and then
to give birth. To accept the shadow is therefore to renounce
beauty and to accept sexuality with change and death.

THE SPECULAR IMAGE AND PREGNANCY

The image we have been speaking of is none other than the
specular image constructed at the mirror stage. Maybe there
wasn't 'jubilation' for woman then, because what happened
for her was not simply 'assumption' or construction from the
'orthopedic' image, but rather **solicitation** [**captation**]. The
girl steps into the mirror and doesn't come out. Contrary to
what happens for the boy, this ego ideal that her mother sees
is her. When will she get herself back? Upon the arrival of
Prince Charming? We do not think that Prince Charming has
the power to wake her up from her dream. Something else is
needed and someone else. The pregnant woman is deformed.
But the alteration of her image, real alteration, still wouldn't
be sufficient to disenchant woman and make her pass into the
real, if she wasn't able, for some other reason, to renounce her
ego ideal. In fact, she lets go of it cheerfully and incautiously,
because, full and fulfilled as she is and momentarily without
anxiety, she thinks she can afford to. She thinks she finally
has something like the penis inside her; her desire for man is
satisfied. It is Tolstoy, in *The Kreutzer Sonata* (1889), who
speaks of these young Russian girls to whom their mothers put
the final touches to turn them into husband traps, and who,
at their first pregnancy, suddenly, completely and definitely
renounce all seduction. The decoy no longer has any use, nor
does the image.

Upon her entry into the mirror – into the specular image – the girl forgets at once her first emotions from the so-called anal and oral stage and from an even more archaic stage. When entering the mirror she lets go of who she was, like another skin. It is no doubt of this forgetting, without repression, that Michèle Montrelay speaks (1970). But it is necessary to insist on the fact that it is the loss of the subject that could have taken place – a loss that happens for the benefit of the imaginary ego ideal. Castration being thus avoided, a swing is instituted between the death of the subject and imaginary existence, leaving no other alternative than mysticism at the level of being: a false mysticism in any case, for woman only swings between the illusory being of the mirror and the non-being of the broken mirror.

If, therefore, pregnancy is a narcissistic crisis ending in pseudo-delusion and depression, it is not only because the ego ideal, the specular image, is massively altered, putting to the test the she-narcissus who wants to remain the same, unchanging and outside of time (losing, what's more, the possibility of also 'stopping' time, as she says). It is above all the fact that, having lost her anxiety, she can afford to let the repressed, or rather the forgotten from before the mirror stage, re-emerge. An emergence facilitated by a return to the very first identification with the mother, if one can use the word identification to define this archaic bond.

In place of the luminous double of the specular image, a shadow moves in, the obscure maternal double. The subject, then, allows the mirror to dull, to become leaden. The 'mask of pregnancy' [masque de la grossesse], these brown spots which cover the forehead and sometimes the whole face, would be nothing else. Aided by this mask, behind the veil, a mutation is in operation. Woman becomes other; the daughter she was becomes a mother. This is the metaphorical meaning of the 'mask of pregnancy'.

'I sleep through my pregnancy,' I was told. Similarly, a character in Faulkner sleeps, stumbling on the road at the end of which she knows she is going to give birth and will then sleep her last sleep. Who is it that gives birth then? It certainly is not 'I'. Deciding to have a child is a deception quite in conformity with the ideology of the new Woman; but the child isn't the product of a decision; even when there was a decision: the child who is born is never the child who had been decided. There is no common measure between the two orders of decision and of childbirth.

If it happens that the woman sleeps through her pregnancy, the birth of the child wakes her up in any case, and sometimes too brutally: she then prefers delusion to wakefulness.

She has already been awakened once before. I would like to locate here this first time which is always mythical, since there is no absolute beginning: it is an important moment in the life of the girl: puberty. There happens, with the coming of menstruation, something like a sudden passage to the state of womanhood. The daughter is no longer the reflection of the mother; she is no longer like the mother. Suddenly, it is the mother who becomes like her, the daughter, a woman; a real woman. She feels her for the first time in her reality as a woman, very close in her flesh, subject to the same organic laws. The daughter, then, knows her mother who becomes untouchable for her. It is a general fact of clinical observation and of ordinary observation: 'Suddenly one evening when we were taking our usual walk, I couldn't hold her arm. . . When I came back from boarding school, I couldn't kiss her and I haven't kissed her since. . . I couldn't touch her; yet she didn't repulse me, no. . .' (cf. Mary Barnes (1971), who says that she wants to love and adore her mother, but cannot go near her).

What happens there is not of the order of repulsion, of jealousy. It is a question of sacred horror. The emptiness which follows is such that the daughter has no other recourse than homosexuality, that is to say another woman, but one who is allowed; or else her father. In both cases, there is a change of object. Love for the father may, in any case, combine with homosexuality; but it may also get the better of it. And if love for the father wins, it may either, after failing, bring the daughter to love another man, or it may remain and trigger a mystical crisis. In any case homosexual love is liable to provide the necessary relay after the break and to allow the daughter, equally, to love men.

This is what an analysand expressed clearly: from the day when, during a trip in a faraway country with a different language, she had dared touch 'the rather large breast of a

woman' in the course of a quite explicit homosexual relation,
she had been able – and right afterwards – 'to be a woman
for men'. She did say 'touch'. It was a question of touching;
not of milk. And the stranger was not her mother and it is as
a stranger that she allowed the young woman to make that
contact.

Phyllis Chesler's argument (1972) seems to us very well
founded; she wants to reconcile woman with woman and sees
the happiness of the heterosexual couple passing through
female homosexuality and even mother-daughter incest. Re-
conciling woman with woman: woman was indeed saving up
too much detestation for herself!

But still, one needs to recognize, under this abdication of
one's own gaze for the benefit of the gaze of the other, an irre-
ducible submission: submission to a law which governs the
very intersubjective relation. As for the politicization of the
problem, we cannot subscribe to it, nor can we follow Phyllis
Chesler when she goes as far as forecasting and preparing
for a time when 'the myth and the reality of the sacrifice of
woman (and of man) will perhaps cease to be. . .' This time is
expected to come about 'when intra-uterine reproduction will
cease or when this function will no longer be assigned to one
of the two sexes'. The remark, with its Marxist connotations,
gives a clue as to Phyllis Chesler's thinking: 'Which will
come about,' she adds with a lot of confidence, 'when women
are able to control the means of production and reproduction'.

When the relays are lacking, the narcissistic passion maintains the adolescent in a suicidal climate, often unacknowl-
edged, even denied by close relatives, but of which it can
be said that it is never absent in the young girl. Where else,
indeed, could her long narcissistic sleep lead her?

The pubertal break, therefore, is decisive and sends the
daughter back to her usual recourse: the saviour-father, at
the same time as the son is struggling with that same father.
However, this break is already the repetition of a former
break, the one which had thrown the girl into the mirror; it is
up to the father, on this occasion as well, to free her from this
devouring spell. But if one easily sees what is the mechanism

through which the daughter goes from mother to father, it is less easy to see how penis envy arises in her.

It would seem that she desires as the absolute Other the one who is neither her mother nor herself: he occupies, for her, the opposite pole. But the opposition is already of a symbolic order, since the girl has at least two trump cards in her game and she plays them. On the other hand, the father is the one to whom the mother turns as well, the one this mother needs to find her **jouissance**. He is therefore the one who has the power. If accidentally the girl has a glimpse of a penis – a fact which is contingent in itself – it then becomes the sign of the phallus. From then on, she can have a representation of the phallus, just as the boy does, through the penis; the only difference being, however, that she doesn't possess the organ as a part of herself. She only has a clitoris; she then hopes for a 'real penis' and expects it from the father. She expects it like a gift. Quite obviously, she will never be given it. If the penis of the boy is assured of a satisfying development, the same is not true of the clitoris. We did find, in a highly specialized book, the description of unusually developed clitorises in homosexual women belonging to a sect of quasi-religious fervour, whose particularity was that 'the sexual part which is called clitoris swells to such proportion that they can use it as a priapus in the act of love' (*La secte des Anandrynes*, 1952); but the important word in this text is the word '**as**'.

I am thinking of the screen-memory (or fantasy, I am not sure) of an analysand, convinced that when she was very small her father had brought her a gift ('a woman cannot love the person who is not able to give presents', says Gina Lombroso in *L'âme de la femme* ['the soul of woman'] (1924)); she didn't understand the meaning of the gift: it was a pot-stand [**dessous de plat**] in blue earthenware. What could a small child do with a pot-stand? It would have been an absurd gift. And yet, thirty years later, she was still wondering. Afterwards, this pot-stand had been used by the family; by the family indeed; by her mother maybe. The father having been killed in the war when the child was three or four, the blue pot-stand had remained as such in her memory, accompanied by an enormous disappointment. This same analysand whom we shall call Philiberte (ϕ + berte or **perte** – loss) was sensitive to the touch of the turgid penis under the rough cloth

of the fly, but she couldn't touch or see a penis in the flesh,
especially flaccid; she was equally very sensitive to the touch
of a firm breast. It is clear that she could not get over the gift
she had not been given – of a paternal phallic object which
the breast could later replace, but of which she demanded in
any case that it should never be soft.

This gift from the father, the phallus, woman expects it,
therefore, until her distant pregnancy. It is thus clear that the
child cannot be said to be the product of the sexual desires of
its parents (even though it is the result of the coitus) and that
one does not go so easily from two (two parts or two beings?)
to three.

FROM TWO TO THREE

The same analysand who said she didn't know how two and
two made four, Anne-Marie, acknowledges much later in
her analysis that she has a 'twin-like' relationship with her
husband. She often speaks of a double monster, minotaur,
centaur, sphinx, Siamese twins, and ends up with her snake
phobia, as they represent for her animals with two similar
extremities: sex/mouth. In a dream, she makes love with
Xavier sex to mouth and mouth to sex, or mouth to mouth and
sex to sex. In a very old dream, a nurse was removing a piece
of flesh from the sex and grafting it onto her mouth.

As for Philiberte, she spontaneously couples people; not
that she actually confuses them. But, if she sees only one of
them in the street or any other public place, she doesn't know
which of the two is standing there, unexpectedly, in front of
her. A minor feature is enough to cloud the issue: spectacles,
a beard, the height; or even some fortuitous circumstance
which has for ever associated the two people in her mind.
Philiberte is not fooled by this spontaneous 'twinning'. She
will occasionally laugh about it, and easily return each to
their respective identity . . . if only to make the same mistake
again immediately afterwards. Equally, she confuses the two
notes of a musical chord into a single sound. She was very
disappointed, in school, to fail her music dictations as soon
as a chord arose in a melody. No one understood the reason
for the failure, neither her teacher, nor her school friends,

nor herself, such was her reputation for infallibility in the matter; did they not say that she had an 'absolute ear'? 'I am obsessed with the triad,' she concluded. Philiberte found in her brother, scarcely older than herself, a double as perfect as the chord, which also made her a prisoner.

She does not have the privilege of this arithmetic symptom. Anne-Marie tells me a dream in the following way: 'The number 2 again: 2 horsemen, a red one and a grey one; the whole problem was to go **between** the two without being knocked over and kicked.' She is the same person who said that she didn't know how 'to locate herself **between** a couple' (cf. chapter 1 on the blood fable). Once she declared: 'I am thirty; in thirty years, I shall be sixty', in a tone of voice which showed how important this discovery was for her.

No doubt woman has to be double, in order to divide into two during childbirth. It is the Russian dolls syndrome, one containing the other in both senses of large and small.

A woman abandoned by her mother at birth has sometimes the greatest difficulty in accepting maternity. It is the case of the novelist Irene Monesi (1966) who admits shamelessly to being an actual child murderer and who writes horrifying novels in order to destroy all maternity for ever.

The two bodies, the body and its double, are the body of the pregnant woman and the foetus, as well as the body of the mother of the pregnant woman and her own. Pregnancy massively brings back the memory of the first couple and with it this archaic so-called 'concentric' libido (cf. Béla Grunberger quoted by Montrelay above, p. 33) as opposed to a phallocentric one. Hence this profusion, this proliferation of fantasies during pregnancy, lived in a kind of sleep or lethargy. So that pregnancy may be compared to a long sleeping cure or a day dream cure where the forgotten would resurface at last. Woman, in a kind of repetition where she merges with her own mother, can then have a representation of what she has lost. At the point of giving birth, she often calls her mother, whom she finally joins, beyond what I have called the pubertal break.

But the repetition may be without solution. Compromised by the failure of the delusion of maternal omnipotence at the time of childbirth, the entry into the real only succeeds on condition that the child is recognized; that is to say, if the

woman, instead of being sucked into the abyss left gaping by the ancient loss of her mother and presently by the delivery of the child, accepts this loss and 'enjoys the new representation that she has of it' (cf. Montrelay, op. cit.). Delivery is then the exact opposite of abortion, such as the process of it was described. In the opposite case, the child does not manage to exist for its mother: one kills the other ('Le meurtre de l'enfant' ['the murder of the child'] in *Scilicet*, 1973).

Through her difficulty in entering the symbolic register defined by the position of the third party, woman comes to wish for the death of the newcomer, this stranger; or that of the husband; she attempts thus to maintain herself in the register of the double. It happens that the husband, jealous of the child, also wishes to kill him. This wish for murder is fiercely denied in the cultural expression of all societies; but it is enough to see the children's cemeteries which cover the hill of Carthage to note that some societies were able to camouflage the murder of the first born, at least, in a ritual. The first born was no doubt the child owed to the deity, in payment of the debt. But the religious ritual covers over, perhaps, a simple inadmissible wish for murder. Unless it sanctifies it and thus allows the murderers to live their murder.

Women analysands speak this wish in a direct way: 'It's him or me'; 'if he is born, I'll die'; 'I'm going to be destroyed'; 'he feeds on my blood'; 'he devours me'; 'I'm afraid to die; they say that they save the mother.' After the birth, the mother feels 'completely eaten up'. 'The child suckles and exhausts me.' 'At night, he prevents me from sleeping.' The mother dreams that she loses him, that she forgets him. During the day, she has the feeling of 'wasting her life'. One of them says that since the birth of her son (who is thirteen months), she has been dreaming at least three times a week that he lies in bed between his parents, suffocating.

It is true, literally, that the child kills his parents, and vice versa. There is no ambivalence in the feeling, but contradiction between **love**, Eros, which wants one and hates the other, and **desire** which is desire of the Other. The contradiction is lived at the level of being: there is a radical impossibility; a fundamental contradiction, in living love and desire. And that which man lives through the love of woman, she lives with the child, or they are both killed by it; the child knows very well that all that is left for him is to save his skin.

In order that a 1 emerge from this mother-child continuum, in order to go from 2 to 3, it is necessary that the extra 1 break the continuum and lock into the chain, a bit like a new word entering into a language which is nevertheless complete. And for that, it is necessary that another factor intervene – or it has been necessary that it intervened. And indeed the word factor can be taken literally [**facteur** also carries the meaning 'postman'].

It is not true that there existed in the world, before the child came, an empty place for him to fill up: other than, quite obviously, the place dug by desire. But this place remains gaping and the world has a hole in it afterwards as it had before. As for his place, the child will violently make it for himself. In order to observe that he does not have it, it is enough to watch an eldest dilated in a family space imaginarily organized for him, when the second child comes to collapse the edifice. The eldest wants to erase this second child, that's all there is to it. He doesn't want him to exist. As the second one insists on living, it is war. No education has ever succeeded in erasing this rivalry. And yet, each makes his place, which is not the expected one. The father should have something to say about that. But, at first, out of the game, without finding anything to say or do, he seeks refuge, so that he may still intervene, in an identification with the other sex.

THE SEX CHANGE [LE CHANGE DE SEXE]

My essential hypothesis was and indeed remains the **sex change**. I have already explained the use of this term (see pp. 12-13). It is quite foreign to Hoffmansthal's tale, which is much too idealistic. Let us start again from Freud (1917): 'In the wish for a baby, an anal-erotic and a genital impulse ("envy for a penis") converge.' As Anne-Marie clearly explained, the delivery is truly expulsion and, if there is orgasm, it is opposed to vaginal orgasm, for 'the vagina swallows'. She added: 'The expulsion had to be explained to me in antenatal classes.'

For her, expulsion was anal expulsion; and besides, shortly

before giving birth, she dreamt that she was defecating, nicely and calmly, next to her mother-in-law, on a balcony.

When I had an orgasm, it was by chance, when I felt like peeing and kept it in; it was a clitoral orgasm. . . But it happens outside; with the vagina, it happens inside; but the women from the women's movement say that it is to please men. . . The man's penis enters, whereas I rather feel the orgasm as pushing out. But I don't know how to push from the vagina.

In any case, delivering a child is 'pushing', and it sometimes provokes an orgasm. An orgasm which is, therefore, the opposite of a vaginal orgasm. The child is lived and experiences itself, as it appears later on, as a faecal sausage; but also as a penis which comes outside and which separates. An analysand spoke of the moment when she felt the child's head stuck between her thighs like a sex, and of the strong illusion she had then of having a penis.

Symmetrically, Ferenczi writes: 'When the increase of tension accumulated within the (male) genital organ propels the head . . . it can be said in some way, that it gives birth.'

There is, therefore, a possible equivalence: male sexual act = female delivery, with reciprocal substitution, woman having an orgasm like man and man like woman. But a woman who delivers and feels something like a penis between her legs, also feels it detaching itself, necessarily. Can it be said that she enjoys the division? As for man, he doesn't lose his penis. That to which he attaches himself, to let go of it later, apart from the mother (and in this, girl and boy are in the same boat) is the breast. The penis is not a lost part object for him. He has it and he is afraid of losing it: it is the phallic stage, with the castration which allows him precisely to symbolize the real loss of the mother, which he has repressed; and beyond, another catastrophic, irreparable loss without content. The girl has indeed a clitoris, but it makes her into an impotent being, incapable of penetrating a woman.

She is left with this 'male protest' which goes into symptoms and becomes neurotically symbolized. The Giraffe, who would like to penetrate herself, frequently dreams that she is losing her hair or her teeth, or sometimes both. This loss can equally be loss of the mother or loss of the penis, of which the clitoris is the small-scale model, and the father the large-scale one. There is repression and symbolization there, but symbolization which, at that level, is founded on identification. This penis that she does not have where it should be: the Giraffe shamefully carries it in the shape of the **neck**, that her long hair fortunately hides. If she hears or thinks she hears the word **giraffe** in her classroom, as she is a teacher, this neck blushes violently. (This was reported two years ago; since then the Giraffe's mother died. A few days after her mother's death, the Giraffe told me this dream: 'I touch my mother's head; the head detaches itself: it has to be put back. There is a red necklace around the neck.' The detachable part, here, is the head.) She cannot bear her bare neck; but neither can she bear a collar, a scarf, a touch or an embrace.

'I'm not a woman,' she says. And yet she has a real knack for detecting the man of whom she is afraid. The one that her husband is not. At the moment, this frightening character is incarnated by a very 'rowdy' Spanish teacher. Can it be said that in the absence of a signifier – that neither her father nor her husband can reveal to her, not being 'rowdy' – she becomes delirious when a real man makes her face that which foreclosure has deprived her of, because this real man confirms the foreclosure, just as the meeting with Dr Flechsig made President Schreber delirious (Schreber, 1903)?

This would amount to saying that 'the' woman is psychotic. But structure and pathology are not analogous. Moreover, if she is psychotic, she is not paranoid for all that, but rather subject to depression or even melancholia.

The Giraffe, therefore, marries a sterile man – one who turns out to be sterile – and the couple has no children. She has come full circle. 'If I had a child,' she says, 'I would become a woman'. Now . . . then. . .

The pregnant woman has something in her at last! Which completes her, like a part of herself. But she will lose this part. Before having it she was wandering like a lost soul, seeking it; after delivery it's already over: she no longer has it. The full and perfect image to which her libido had flowed back, crumbles. The delusion of omnipotence collapses; a wish for murder (murder of the child) replaces it sometimes. In ordinary cases this stasis of the libido of which Freud speaks can be observed. There is no longer an object, because there is no longer an image. She doesn't have this child whom it is claimed she has.

It is a patent failure which exposes her to 'a mutilation . . . which will be marked along the weak joins of the fragmented body' as Granoff and Périer say in their 'Recherches sur la féminité ['Research on femininity'] (1964). At that moment, woman has it no longer and she is nothing. After omnipotence, annihilation. The newcomer, the child, is irrevocably the Other. The husband, who meanwhile has become a mother, and is often ill in these trying times, can do little. Sexual intercourse which has been interrupted for a while is not immediately resumed. The new mother speaks of 'fear', of 'repulsion' or simply of absence of desire; and the new father is not always as keen as he claims he is to make love with this lover who has become a mother. She finds herself, therefore, separated from her husband at the same time as she is confronted with emptiness: 'Depression through symbolic lack', as Brigitte Chardin says (1974), except when there is an appropriate intervention, when the mother is in analysis. But, 'if the elaboration of the transference does not allow going beyond its character of resistance towards its character of interpretation of the desire of the Other, the subject remains caught in a position of conflict'.

Amongst the possible outcomes, Brigitte Chardin notes:
— the end of the treatment or the wish for a break;
— an abortion;
— a mastered and competitive delivery.

The more 'wonderful' pregnancy and delivery were, the more difficult the following period is going to be. The word 'competitive' which Brigitte Chardin uses to describe these exploits is quite appropriate. The new mother has most often followed a kind of training, namely antenatal classes. She talks a lot about her abdominal muscles and her breathing.

One of them, back after her delivery, gave this typical account of it: 'Marvellous delivery, like a sporting performance. Wonderful memory. . .' etc.; then: 'Awful awakening; floods of blood . . . tears . . . nightmare . . . husband ill, staying with his mother, therefore absent. . .' And then: 'It's a girl; I was expecting a boy.'

It happens that the husband, for his part, doesn't get over the experience. He remains feminized. It is because in the couple the child replaces the husband who, being no longer of any use, feels rejected, unless he keeps to the role of dry nurse and takes the place of mother alongside his wife. No longer able to have the Other (the Woman), he has indeed become it. He has feminized himself as much as possible. His own way of being a woman, his way of begetting, is to **carry the child** (Tournier, 1967; 1970), not in his stomach of course, although often things happen there, but outside, on his back or in his arms. It is the 'child-carrying' man [**l'homme porte-enfant**], like the hero of Michel Tournier, St Christopher, and all the ancient or modern pederasts.

Feminizing himself, man finds in that instance his only opportunity of acceding to the figure, as Lacoue-Labarthe (1975) says in a commentary on Hegel: 'It cannot be said of the masculine figure that it is, in the most rigorous sense, a figure. Masculinity figures itself with difficulty or, at the limit, can only figure itself by feminizing itself.' We shall return to this point in connection with woman's beauty.

Meanwhile the woman has become a man through vocation; for if the object of her love and of her identification has always been the father, she has herself, paradoxically, become this father during pregnancy. She becomes, in fact, homosexual, to take up Lacan's spelling. The sex change is consummated.

The channelling of the libido towards the child – which can go, with everybody's blessings, as far as erotomania, at the expense of the husband and of sexual intercourse – is the outcome of the old feminine dream of fulfilment and completion: she is a man since she has the phallus (the child) and she is a woman since she is a mother. She therefore is **everything**, if not all, to take up Lacan's expression once more. And, as they say: motherhood has transformed her!

In short, no sooner has woman come out of the narcissism of childhood and adolescence, and succeeded in loving man, when she goes through a new acute narcissistic crisis, during pregnancy. After which, two paths are open to her to refind the real: the man and the child. The path that leads to the child remains, however, strongly narcissistic and perpetuates as such the mother-child relationship. The other path, the one that goes through man, crosses it. It happens that a woman has her first vaginal orgasm after her first or even her second delivery. It is at least an old popular belief that childbirth cures the frigid woman. What about this **jouissance** happening at last? It signifies perhaps that the failure of narcissism during delivery has had an effect. If it is true, as Granoff and Périer write, that 'all love carries castration within it', maternal love does too. And woman, as every speaking being, can only find **jouissance** through castration and language. It seemed to us that woman invents her own way for herself in following this double path, an often difficult and contradictory one since the lover cannot be mother, nor the mother lover.

When she refuses castration and pretends to be everything, woman of course becomes mad. When she is not everything, she still runs the risk of being double.

Michèle Montrelay says that she loves herself in her body, as if it were the body of an other. Indeed, the Giraffe, for example, dreams that she is a man and that she makes love with herself. But it is barely a dream, for she also says – and we think that any woman could say it – that she would like to be a man 'to feel what he feels when he makes love with her/woman'. Paraphrasing Valéry's *La jeune Parque* (1917), following Lacan's commentary on it, we would say that she felt herself feeling herself. Lacan adds: 'The "I saw myself seeing myself" has its full meaning when it is a question of femininity. But we are not there yet.' That was in 1964.

In order to feel herself, why does she need to use the sex of man, precisely that of man? And what is the use in question?

The Giraffe frequently makes love in her dreams, although she sleeps in the same bed as her husband and they have frequent sexual intercourse. In short, she makes love by herself, in one way or another, and we would say that she masturbates, if this term could have any meaning when applied to a woman.

We have made pregnancy and delivery into something equivalent for woman to the sexual act for man. In this matter, it is quite clear that the misunderstanding continues. Man seeks the Other in woman; but he only finds the object (a), cause of his desire. He finds mostly his mother, the sexual act awakening in him an archaic libido, preceding sexualization and sexual difference. He loses his sex in it. As for woman, she seeks the omnipotent paternal phallus in man and the sexual act, and she only finds a penis, subject to failure, subject at least to detumescence. In order to preserve the paternal phallus, she falls back onto the maternal function and becomes herself phallic. It is the very process of change. She is no longer castrated, if she ever was!

WOMAN AS SPEAKING BEING

But what then is the value of her speech? Shall we say that woman is mute or that she only speaks to make noise? No, there cannot be two human races. Man and woman are speaking beings. And Lacan, in one of his schemas (1972-3), starts from the speaking being before finishing off men and women. It is true that woman seems to escape **symbolic** castration. She is actually more knowledgeable about **real** deprivation, for which she compensates with a wish for and a fantasy of totality. We are in agreement here with Michèle Montrelay according to whom 'woman does not know repression'. But that is true – and she says so specifically – of the woman, not of a woman, who is always partly man as well.

Woman has a clitoris which, as we said, can make a man out of her (albeit castrated) and allows her, at least, to identify with a man. The bisexuality of the foetus up to the eighth week makes of the sexual difference a phenomenon of differentiation: the sexes therefore retain the **capacity** for each other, denying thereby the work of subjective (signifying) appropriation of the sex. According to which side one looks – and it is therefore simply a question of point of view – if woman is whole, the something in man is extra; if man is whole, it is woman who has something less. One can say that differentiation operates through a something less or more. But it is always the same thing, which is for ever being asked for, given and lost, always fallaciously, without ever achieving the exchange.

The gap is irreparably instituted when the something more is incarnated in the male sexual organ, which allows man symbolically to bring into play only a part of himself, whereas woman continues to swing wholly between her double and nothingness, refusing symbolic castration.

The real deprivation of a part of herself – the child – becomes once more imaginary frustration, when it awakens the loss of this other part of herself, her mother, from a fantasy of totality. Now, through this oscillation from imaginary to real, the **symbolic** can be instituted, as we saw, owing to the lifting of the archaic repression through childbirth on the one hand, and the encounter with man in coitus on the other. Woman can choose one or the other path or one and the other path. But both are useful. For, on the one hand, enjoying man as the Other – the father – she easily becomes an hysteric if she doesn't have a child. And, on the other hand, if she is only mother, she does not come out of her narcissism and remains parapsychotic because she misses the Other. If she has not known and loved her real father, she is in danger of never knowing orgasm; and if she has not known that she loved her mother, she runs the risk of not being able to have a child.

Man – if it wasn't for his wish to participate in creation like a woman – would be, is, more autonomous. He has every opportunity of playing with the object (a). Woman has less of a margin and less humour. But she can also say to man: 'Keep talking. . .' He replies, it is true: 'You castrate me and you're a pain in the neck.'

And yet it is woman, the mythical being who incarnates the Other for man, whom he questions, as the place of truth, source of life and origin, which she obviously is not. He questions her, as Dante did Beatrice, Socrates did Diotimes, and Oedipus did the Sphynx.

When she replies, it is as Pythia, as a witch, as a clairvoyant, as a mystic. She tells what the voices tell her. She does not speak in her own name. Perhaps she is not a subject. Guardian of graves, as we know she has been since Antigone, she stands at the gates of life and death; and from there she hears something.

Shall we say that it speaks perhaps, but that she does not speak? No. It would be too wonderful. What is true is that, denounced as the subject that she is not, offering herself as an evidence of lure, she, as a result, saves on a great deal of false certainties.

As for man he only speaks of her and for her. Inasmuch as she speaks like him, she steals his speech and castrates him. She is a being of violence, indeed; she doesn't recognize the law, even if she submits to it. The divine law of Antigone is barely what authorizes her to rebel against human law. Woman steals speech, penis and child. When she steals literally (in shops) it is on impulse. This problematic of theft is a response to that which is less in woman and of which she is deprived, and to the fallacious gift that she expects from the father.

There is a discourse that man, unless he were to imitate her, cannot steal from her: that of begetting. It can rightly be said: discourse, since it is a question of a chain of terms. Certainly the child is at first (perhaps) conceived as the symbol of the unity of the couple, and often the proof (which would otherwise be missing) of that unity. Actually, it is rather expelled or lost as a part object, as we saw; and itself in being born abandons its envelope, the placenta (This, 1975), and more structurally what makes it be born, what makes it be. Rather than metaphor and assumption of the other, the child is then metonymy, and doomed as such to reproduce endlessly. It remains that it is not begot by the mother only. Fortunately – for man's intervention in the sexual act and its sequels have the effect of allowing the child, whatever its sex, to accede to the symbolic world and to escape the fatality of the double. It is then instituted as a subject and takes up the genealogical chain, for a while under threat of being cut off by parental narcissism.

The more specific question of the psychoanalyst is to wonder if women are analysable. What they say, according to Michèle Montrelay who follows Freud, is so transparent, so close to the unconscious, that it discourages interpretation and makes intervention useless.

I do not think so. When the woman analysand speaks – pouring out or almost mute – one can say that in her it speaks psychotically, metonymically, rather than neurotically and metaphorically. Now, psychotic and metonymic is also how President Schreber's discourse appears. One might say that woman hears voices. For the psychoanalyst, it is a golden speech, consequently. When there is repression and not foreclosure, and repression is lifted, woman speaks like man and is analysed in the same way.

The divergences noted in these pages are the fact of femininity, not of women, and they may recognize themselves there or not. It is these divergences which institute the sexual difference, the possibility of coitus and begetting, as well as the impossibility of sexual relation as 'rapport'; an impossibility which is the very condition of the language of man **and** woman. There is the speaking being, and man and woman signifiers, which this speaking being plays, precisely in order to speak. It is appropriate to refer here to the schema in which Lacan figures sexual disparity (1972-3).

$\exists x \quad \overline{\Phi x}$ $\forall x \quad \Phi x$	$\overline{\forall x} \qquad \Phi x$

The father of the primal tribe, as the term which posits the exception, denies castration (φx); there exists therefore at least one; which is written: $\exists x \overline{\varphi} x$. But for every man ($\forall$), there exists a value of x such as one can write $\forall x \varphi x$: it is the phallic function. For part of the speaking beings ($\forall$), this function may be denied or not (up to now I have been following word for word the reading suggested by Lacan himself for this schema).

I shall now inscribe the child in E (it is my own addition to the schema which, in any case, is incomplete here) at the point of junction of $\mathcal{S} \to a$ and of the $a \to \varphi$. Then, drawing a dotted line E . . $\to S(\overline{A})$, I shall force the child into the mythical line of the Great Ancestor and into the symbolic lineage of the father. But first we shall make of him the product of the junction of two desires.

What does the product of desire signify? Let us return to a couple at the time of conception. They want a child or they don't. In either case, the child who is born has no common measure with this desire. And, firstly, there are at least two desires, that of the father and that of the mother. These two desires determine a sexual relation based on lure since the desire of the Other is reduced there to the assimilation of the (a). There results a foreign body, product of ingestion and assimilation, and a rejected and expelled left over. The child therefore is this product and this left over, destined to occupy a place in the world. The world being full, it was not an empty place, except, as we saw, in the imaginary space of the parents.

In so far as the desire to have a child replaces sexual desire as such (desire of the Other), it is the child who becomes the object (a), on the condition that it stays the Same and becomes at the same time the Other, for the parent carrier of that desire or both. An impossible condition.

The child will have to recover from this status of product, or left over or object (a), in order to become entitled to his own desire to exist. It is the Oedipal crisis. Analysis describes the very process of releasing at the end of which the subject speaks.

But the child does not speak and with good reason.

Of course it screams at birth; it cries; it is looked at, soon it smiles, then it babbles. Feeding and body care, like the scream, the tears, the gaze and the smile are already language. In that sense the child speaks and is spoken to, otherwise how would it begin to speak one day? What needs to be remembered here, is not that he speaks in some way already; but that he does not speak yet, for that is what defines him as an in-fant.

Moreover, following Jakobson's work, the scream and the babble can be taken as a prelanguage, followed by a period of aphasia, itself followed by the appearance, at around three, of proper language, all of a sudden. This language, more rigid and poorer than babble, is the common language, and it does not directly come out of babble. The mutism of the child occupied with absorbing the common language marks a break, an empty time during which the child renounces the plenitude of his idiom which is, according to Dante, the language of his nurse and, according to Jakobson, a psychotic

type of language. Being born into language and into the
symbolic order is therefore renouncing a full and private
language.

The mystery of the appearing of the child, elsewhere, in
another place, as an external material body, remains whole.
Certainly, a work is always defined by its characteristic of
material body having its own organization; but it is equally
defined as what is left over. From a detachable object, the
child will have to move to an individual counting for one.

If they want him to be a masterpiece, it is worse still.
He is done for: he will never be one thing or another, man
or woman. It is the fate of children of narcissistic parents.
(For, of course, the father can be narcissistic too.) The child
is obliterated from the start as image and alienated in his
function of mirror in relation to the parents. The object
(a) finds here its perfect illustration, since it is always of the
register of the Same: whom will this child resemble? And it is
the kill. Narcissism being a universal given, every child will
have to free himself from these forced identifications; for
being a child, not speaking, is participating as object (a) in the
parental narcissistic organization. To the very extent of this
participation, the language that is learnt will be echolalic.

If the parents have not wanted the child, to the extent of
wishing it dead, it is destined to survive as a redundant object
deprived of speech. It is the fate of the mute child. It is a kind
of abortion.

This paradoxical status of the child who does not speak
is equally that of man himself, whose access to speech is not
natural but who, on the contrary, passes through a series of
défilés [see glossary] each of which includes a loss.

But, finally, he – the man after the child – speaks. The child
who does not speak, precisely for the reason that he has been
conceived to serve and must not count as one, illustrates what
the schema brings to the fore through the in and out drawing
of the two desires.

The evidence of the line, however, doesn't facilitate things
for whoever might claim to understand. One must not understand too quickly, says Lacan. There is no such risk. But
the warning is of value mainly as a statement of principle.
To whoever believes they understand from the start and

completely, it can be stated that they are mistaken, from the very fact that meaning is not fixed: this meaning is only ever that which the present language gives to the schema. It is represented by the horizontal stroke which separates the proposition concerning the speaking being above, from the sexual meaning below: man/woman. But it is appropriate to leave an area of wavering.

It is absolutely necessary to start from a general proposition, namely – as we have said – from the speaking being; not from man and woman already separated, for that would make them into two entities. Hence it would become quite impossible to conceive the **one**, except in positing a god through whom love would be defined. For the sexual characteristic is already an attribute. There is an incompatibility between the Being and the One, said Plato's Parmenides: as soon as the Other is posited, a quality is attributed to him, here a sexual one. Thus the sexual difference can be posited as exemplary and even fundamental in the range of differences. But if this male or female quality is assimilated to something which would be of the order of the universal, one ends up with this absurdity that two One are created which are different. And it is not possible either to start from the absolute, universal One; for from this One, there would never result Two.

Luce Irigaray (1974b) criticizes Freud for scotomizing femininity: 'The pleasure obtained from touch, caress, the half opening of the labia, of the vulva, simply doesn't exist for Freud, all these organs apparently lacking male parameters.' The title: '*The blind spot within an old dream of symmetry*' insists on this criticism of scotomization.

There is no doubting the fact that male and female organs are anatomically different. It is destiny, says Freud. But here again, it is a question of inscription, that is to say of language.

So man and woman are equipped with different sexual organs, even though genetics are far from categorical on this point; and nature in its variations even less so. But the essential is to show that these differences are taken or taken up at the level of language, and with the sole aim of maintaining the sexual difference. (As is shown by the apologue of the toilets told by Lacan which we shall pick up later, see pp.54–5.) Freud is much more revolutionary than Luce Irigaray, in spite of appearances, when he posits a fundamental bi-sexuality and a signifying differentiation. What concerns the psychoanalyst, in any case, is the 'subjective declaration of belonging to a sex' (*Scilicet* 4, 1973).

It is then necessary to start from a mythical region, or an abstract one if one wishes, which would be situated beyond history; that is the one which is represented above the stroke in the schema, whereas below humankind is represented in its history. In order to define the region above, we may take up the words of Pierre Legendre (1974): 'Ideal and absolute space where dogmatic propositions are invented, a mathematic-like space which doesn't know history; radically antecedent and not constituted, where we are separated from any speaking being.' But where we posit them as such.

In this space a law may indeed be exposed and inscribed, and it is this one: 'There exists at least one for whom there exists a value of x such as φ of x is denied. (Which is written $\bar{\varphi}$x.) Which allows every speaking being ($\forall$x) to posit φx.' It is the phallic function which is thus defined. The speaking being draws from it the ability to speak because of the impossibility of the sexual 'rapport', which if it were possible would sign the death of desire.

This law can be stated as its opposite (on the right of the schema), namely: 'For a number of speaking beings, on condition precisely of being **this not all**, of allowing no universality, it is allowed to posit oneself or not in φx.'

With the beginning of history, which in any case is arbitrarily fixed, the speaking being posits itself as sexual, that is to say separate. He says I, and I is firstly: not you. He names himself therefore, as separate or barred. It is the barred subject ($). He needs the other to say I; to say it to him. The other par excellence for man, is woman, and vice versa. That is why sexual difference is taken, quite rightly, as the fundamental model of all difference.

$, which signifies the subject, has an absent signified which is this very bar. One can also say: insofar as he is sexed (split, but beware of the myth of unity of Aristophanes!) man desires that which he does not have, the Other. But he only finds his imaginary fellow [**semblable**], the (**a**). Which is written $\$\Diamond A$. We know this formula of fantasy.

All of this is inscribed on the left of the schema, whereas on the right a number of speaking beings are characterized through finding their **jouissance** in the ετερος, in the Other, S(Ⱥ), of which it has been said that it was the father. Why name the category on the right **women** and the category on the left **men**? It is time to recall the apologue of the toilets mentioned above (Lacan, 1966).

Two children, brother and sister, facing each other, look each from their own perspective, as the train slows down, at two identical cubicles on the platform and read the two different sets of initials above the door: H and D [**Hommes** and **Dames**: Gentlemen and Ladies]. The distinction of the toilets – for they are toilets – is founded only on the difference of initials and on the separation of the sexes which this difference commands, a separation which is demanded by custom and expressed through language. They are therefore isolating cubicles: to each sex his own. That is the only thing which distinguishes them. It is clear, here, that the signified are not located somewhere in the toilets: the H is a signifier which represents the subject (the little girl) who reads: **men**, for another signifier, the D which the little boy reads.

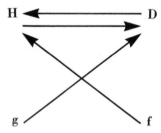

For the M would have no meaning in itself. It could indeed just as well signify the name of the town, if it was not joined to the W. It would continue to have no meaning of town or sex or whatever, if a subject was the only one to see it. This is a completely gratuitous hypothesis. The same goes for the words man and woman in the Lacanian schema.

Word or initials take on meaning only through the fact that another subject sees the other in a criss-crossing process: the signifying terms, here, are coupled for the convenience of the argument, but we know that their series is infinite.

Which doesn't mean that these words **man** or **woman** are entirely arbitrary, nor that they could be reversed. Certainly, they are in no way justified or authenticated by etymology. There was no original religious language which would be the guarantee of the meaning of words. The 'proof through etymology' does not hold, as Jean Paulhan demonstrated some years ago (1953). But from the moment history began, the 'nodal points' have been functioning in such a way that the individual cannot arbitrarily handle a language.

If we place ourselves below the bar, we are already inside a certain meaning, within a full history which is ours and which is founded on the sexual difference, and there is henceforward a word to say man and a word to say woman. **Language and sexual difference are contemporary**. One founds the other. That is why, at the start of the game, Lacan lays his cards on the table: men's side/women's side. To return to the apologue, there is a kind of disfunctioning in the couple, expressed through the criss-crossing of the toilets, as long as we do not forget, certainly, that the train is slowing down, but more particularly that it is still going and will start up again, all of which determines a certain delay, a certain interval in the mechanics of the crossing looks. It could be objected that the brother and the sister would only have to look at each other to learn everything about their respective sex. But, precisely, that is what they do not do, because of a 'horror of knowing' as Lacan says. Man does not want to know. He goes around the houses a lot.

So then, what is agreed to be called The woman – inasmuch as she exists – has her **jouissance** in the Other, whereas the cause of man's desire is the disappointing (*a*); if one figures the two desires by the arrows, one sees that they are crossing, they do not go in each other's direction. Besides, woman also desires the phallus; hence a second arrow above.

In summary, therefore, the schema can be read as follows:

For every man ($\forall$), there exists a value of x ($\forall$x) for which φx is posited. It is the phallic function.

For a number of speaking beings ($\forall$), that is to say not every man, it is allowed for each one to posit himself in φx or not to be a part of it.

Underneath, the sexual partner is inscribed, on man's side,

$, supported by the φ as signified. It is the subject barred by his lack. It is only through the intermediary of the object (a) that he reaches his sexual partner, the Other.

On the contrary, woman situated in the (a) finds her **jouissance** in the Other: S(Å) which is the father. But it also happens that she desires. 'That is why she is not all,' says Lacan.

Whereas man is easily the plaything of fantasy and can only stop loving a woman through loving another one, unless he fixates onto another fetish object; woman's vocation for her part is to love in the symbolic register or to **love**, period, and to love one man only (the play of the four fathers being played only in childbirth). Generally man seeks to escape from this love. He feels caught, trapped, eaten up by the woman who loves him. Through preventing him from running after his fantasy, she deprives him of the cause of his desire, the object (a), and she castrates him by becoming for him a mother who fulfils his demand. What about woman then?

She often rushes into two impasses which are expressed for us by two questions:

— is the libido male?

— how can woman have access to symbolic castration?

Before answering them, let us attempt to clear the avenues of these questions.

We have seen the daughter tied to the mother – just as the male baby is – by an archaic anal and oral link; at the time of the mirror stage, this link hampers, in the female baby, the assumption of the subject and favours the formation of an ego ideal at the expense of the real (we speak about the feminine, of course, as an entity, while positing that there is no woman who follows our definitions). If the girl succeeds in speaking earlier than the boy – which is frequent – it is no doubt due to her power of identification; she is **pretty** as a **picture** and you can't be prettier than a picture; she speaks **like** mummy. She is a little woman. We have seen that childbirth allows the woman precisely to represent to herself this archaic loss of the mother and that this very representation opens up for her a possible access to the real. But then has she been sleeping or dreaming until now? And if she awakes sooner, who awakens her from this narcissistic sleep?

Kore-Persephone was picking poppy flowers when Pluto met her and abducted her. Thus the young girl was sleeping in her mother's love; and she was as though raped. Demeter obtained, by dint of complaints, that she be given back to her – periodically given back.

It sometimes happens that the man who rapes the girl is her own father. And if she lets herself be raped, it is no doubt that she desired the phallus in him, if not the penis. She had been desiring it, this phallus, for ever. When, by chance, she happened to see a penis, the desire for the phallus was expressed through penis envy; provided that this penis was invested as liable to be lacking. The only thing is, the woman herself does not lack anything, at least in the sense that she is not liable to be missing any organ, except in the case of symptomatic surgical intervention (cf. below, p. 137).

It is therefore as sign of the difference that she first sees the penis, and secondarily as proof of a lack representing that lost primary object; hence these fantasies of loss that she develops afterwards (hair, teeth, etc.) as substitutes for an imaginarily lost penis. But whereas for the boy the penis is felt as the phallic representative par excellence of a proper lack, the girl is not in the same boat and it is elsewhere (with the father) that she intends to preserve it, so that it may be given to her later. Thus declared – through this gift – as the favourite daughter, she is reassured and pretends to believe that she is no longer exposed to the risk of losing herself. . . It is not in woman's nature to expose herself.

THE IMAGINARY DIVISION

And yet, she speaks and she stands up. And when she gives birth, she shows herself to be having a phallic function which culminates at that point and which she doesn't hold solely by proxy. (Let us say, to lift any apparent contradictions in the use of the word **phallus**, that it can be figured as a monument put in the place of lack which is thus at once denounced and camouflaged.) Furthermore, the clitoris and the breasts are erectile organs which give her pleasure. If they cannot symbolize castration, because they are not threatened with anything, they nevertheless express a properly female phallic function. What about the threat of castration then, which does not bear – as we know – on the real loss of an imaginary object?

The expulsion of the child and the withdrawal of the penis constitute real separations from a real object representing an imaginarily lost part of the female body. But there is a process of contamination with castration properly speaking, aided by the fact that woman has her own phallic organization. The penis becomes for her, as for the man, the symbol of the threatened phallus, whereas the vagina represents the absence of it.

It remains to be explained how this process of contamination takes place. We have seen that the girl loses her mother a second time, when she discovers that her mother loves her father; she then feels not castrated, but negated. In that way she also loses her only recourse: the father. And, like an orphan, she seeks refuge in a frenzied narcissism. She loves herself 'intensely', says Freud. She takes herself as a love object and has the exemplary dream of the Giraffe. This virile, active other may become a persecuting voice. The father is quite powerless to free her from it: it is not the Other she needs indeed, it is a real man, having accepted symbolic castration and equipped with a penis. Or, even, as Freud says, a penis equipped with a man's body.

This other – who is not, for all that, an object (a) – woman has no difficulty in recognizing, when she finds him, because he was already there, constitutively. When it reappears in the shape of the penis or of the child, which move in her with their own movements, she separates from the imaginary other who has become useless; as she will separate, when the time comes, from the penis and from the child. Rather than castration anxiety, woman knows **division** anxiety. She truly lives under the sign of abandonment: mother, father, children, husband, penis, everyone leaves her.

When the penis comes, it is therefore in place of the plug that the imaginary other constituted in respect of the division. Except that this new other who moves with his own movement, indicating thus the presence of another subject, constitutes from then on a love object in the real. The description of the female vaginal orgasm given by Michèle Montrelay illustrates perfectly this moment of revelation. From now on woman symbolizes the imaginary loss of a part of herself by the phallic organ par excellence, the penis. It is female symbolic castration.

Is division, then, the homologue of castration? It is not, if one recalls that symbolic castration can only intervene when set in motion on one's own body. Certainly separation affects woman's body; but it is symbolized in a foreign organ, the penis; and secondarily in the vagina, as receptacle of the penis and possibly symbol of its lack. What woman symbolizes in her own body is therefore secondarily the lack of that which she had not posited the presence of. Thus I would like to call her 'la malcastrée' ['the badly castrated'] using for myself the title of a recent work (Santos, 1973). This twofold process of castration is indeed often maladjusted and leads woman not at all to refuse castration, but on the contrary to experience herself as castrated. She therefore ordinarily remains on this side of imposture as subject. It is pure profit from the viewpoint of truth, if not at the level of daily life. The process of symbolic castration in man would likewise need to be analysed. It would be discovered no doubt that castration is represented in and through the female body and that originally it is lack, break, division, separation from the mother – since the boy is born, just as the girl, from a mother –; and that this process is twofold for him as well.

In summary, the real man, the other one but not the (a) frees the woman from the introjected paternal phallus, as the child frees her from a deathly maternal double. No more blinding sun, no more shadow either; but a possible real. This access to the real, proper to woman, is however not easy for her; not even natural. She is more familiar with impasse than with social sublimation, other than maternal. A recent film (*Jeanne Dielman*, made by Chantal Akerman, 1976) gives a very good account of the impasse as well as of the passage à l'acte. It portrays a woman with eyes which do not see but with a sure hand, sinking into domestic occupations (and never has the word occupation had a fuller sense) until she becomes the best functioning machine in the house. In the afternoon she makes love for money; one must make a living. She functions, absent. A sentence of Gina Lombroso (cf. p.36) came back to me while watching her functioning in that way:

'Woman resembles an electric bell which is lacking an insulator and which not only rings conscientiously at each call, but continues ringing even when it is no longer pressed and you want it to stop.'

Worse still if one intends to alter its programme. Which is what happened to the machine called Jeanne Dielman: a man having gone over the time which was assigned to him between washing up and bathing, the machine started making small mistakes; nothing was done on time any longer, until the day when this very man managed to make her come, in spite of herself. Then coldly, calmly, she killed him. She stuck some scissors in his throat. Was he not sticking his penis 'like a knife' in her body? **Now, she did not want to come.** A refusal of **jouissance**: it does not prevent one from seeming to live closest to the real. Actually, Jeanne Dielman only reached the real in murder. And yet she is an ordinary woman.

The sociologist Seymour Fisher notes, in a survey on female orgasm, that the so-called working-class women or peasant women have less orgasms than educated middle-class women. The wild woman would seem to be a myth. It seems therefore that there isn't a sexual instinct in woman which would allow her to find the penis at the appointed time, this penis not being the natural object of her desire.

The real other, for all that, except for deviance, is not the sole organ, the sole penis (which in this case becomes the fetish object); the penis is not cause of desire either. If the cause of man's desire is the object (a) which woman shows off with a great display of artifice, the cause of woman's desire is the phallus, that is to say that which the penis represents. To the feminine masquerade answers the masculine parade and it is owing to this game of illusionists that they meet at all. That there is no sexual relation does not signify that there is no sexual intercourse and that nothing happens. But only that there is no complementary union of two opposites which could be equated. There is illusion, misdeal: woman pretending to be what she is not and man showing what he does not have.

Thus the division which is immanent in desire makes itself felt through being experienced in the desire of the Other, in that it already opposes itself to the subject being satisfied to present to the Other whatever real he may have, since what

he has is worth no more than what he does not have, for his

demand of love which would want him to be it. (Lacan, 1966)

Thus man makes woman into his phallus and woman makes man into the phallophore, her phallus-carrier.

And yet something happens. After the event, both are changed: certainly that doesn't happen every day, and its not happening doesn't prevent pleasure. But in **jouissance**, something in the real is grasped, which modifies the signifying chains of both. The effect of it can be seen afterwards in their language and their daily life, for each has then something to say or do.

And that is why woman, like man, speaks. And why she is not mute. It remains, and it surely is not a sociological nor a cultural fact that this speech is often difficult, that it is not self-evident.

'Every woman,' writes Hélène Cixous (1975) 'has known the torment of coming to oral speech; the pounding heart, sometimes a fall into a loss of language; the ground giving way; such is the extent of speaking – I would even say opening her mouth in public – being for woman foolhardiness, transgression. A double distress, for even if she transgresses, her speech almost always falls on the deaf masculine ear which only hears in language that which is spoken in the masculine.'

I shall add: especially deaf to the complaint men want to know nothing about, which they cannot bear; and that women bring to the temple, in front of the tabernacle, despite all interdiction, if we are to believe Jacques Hassoun, in order to force men to hear it. 'If I speak, I cry,' a woman analysand says to me.

Indeed, opening her mouth is trying for a woman: what flux, what flow, what breath, what blood is going to escape? Or is it in order to devour that they open their mouth, like Penthesilea?

It happens that man makes the same neurotic confusion between speech and flux or flow. Such is the case of this phobic man, Roi, reported by the psychoanalyst Colette Rouy (1974), who felt the need to vomit the morning of his exams, and sees this need repeating itself to the extent that it interferes with his life. The day before, he had heard his brother tell their mother, in the bathroom, that he was going to get married because his fiancée was pregnant. Since then, the need [les envies] to vomit which he designates simply by 'They' [Elles] persecutes him. 'They' only cease when he speaks, during his courses or his lectures. He therefore has to speak all the time in order not to vomit. Schreber too used to vomit. . . When one thinks that Roi's obsession is to carry a child (he dreams of rescued children) and that he searches for his female double, one can only suppose that he has made a female identification, to say the least.

To go back to woman, certainly she has something to say, whereas often man speaks and says nothing – would say nothing if woman was not there to be questioned. Then who is speaking? Neither; or both.

3

From division to symbolic castration

It remains for me to tell you about the
madness of a reasonable woman, in order to
show you that madness is often nothing else
than reason under a different guise.

Goethe, *Wilhelm Meister's Years of Travel*

USING as a pretext what I was told by a young woman of twenty-one whom I shall call Aucassine, because with her the whole question of the Middle-Ages is evoked, I enter into a domain which one can call, with Phyllis Chesler (1972), that of women's madness.

Here is what Aucassine says: 'I have flashes. They get thicker and thicker. I don't see things or objects any longer. I'm very scared. I don't want it to be noticed. I hold on as long as I can. I hurt everywhere. And then I burst and it's over. I'm empty.'

'. . . Last night I didn't sleep. I remembered a time when I was kissing a boy: our two mouths became like world wide caverns. Very dark. I screamed. I burst my lungs. I said: "I'm dead." What I try to remember is the point when I'm dying. . .'

'. . . I told them that I was a foetus, that my mother had abandoned me. My mother was my friend Monique. I was very thirsty. She put saliva in my mouth . . . when I saw a boy in the bed, I screamed. Then there was the time when I was in hell. I didn't see the walls any more. . .'

Aucassine is not mad. She studies Hebrew; she is already in her second year; she pays for her room by giving lessons to two children for two hours a day; she paints the walls of her room with friends. She lives comfortably and, at least outwardly, reasonably. Besides, she receives generous monthly allowances from her father, a lawyer. Maître Grassier (a name which I always mentally write as **gracié [pardoned]**) is a Protestant and his elder brother is a minister.

Mad or not; perhaps pretending? I do not believe it. But it is not necessary to decide. What she says, she says. I shall, however, call delusion that which is becoming clearer wit some of the following family data. This delusion is precisel a family one as it unfolds around the 'message' which the mother says she has received, with the responsibility to transmit it. Mother's parents were non-believers; the message was therefore received by her, directly from God. She is the **first** touched by grace. In order to transmit the message, she needed no less than twelve children: twelve prophets she had them.

They are grouped in two; the eldest of each couple having studied or studying normally or brilliantly, and the youngest lagging behind. Thus the eldest girl is a lawyer; single mother, she lives with her younger sister, a social worker, equally without a man. Together they bring up their two children. They are both mystics, but not Protestant; they have opted for an oriental religion.

Then come two boys; the eldest is a minister like his uncle; the youngest is a worker, unemployed and alcoholic.

Aucassine is an eldest, of the third couple. She studies Hebrew, as I said, but also English and German. When she was fifteen she loved a German man of twenty-five, whom she calls 'a wise man' or 'a philosopher'. Finally, she writes poems. Her younger sister has just arrived from the country to stay with her in Paris, with a 'message'; a text which was 'dictated' to her and that she must have published urgently. She has already been around the publishing houses in the country. In it she explains her mission; she is Christ and has received the command to save mankind. She spent three days and three nights writing the text without sleep.

The other children are similarly organized in couples, down to the last girl who is decidedly 'apart'. 'She is a baby and she will remain a baby.' This family without any operating men (they are progenitors, but not operators in the work of family structuration) is distributed, as we see, according to a dualistic principle, following a labyrinthine system of

mirrors. All the features characteristic of femininity can be
found in it (inasmuch as one can speak of femininity):

— non-paranoid mysticism: the women have visitations or are possessed;
— poetic gift and writing;
— collective or simply family delusion: the message;
— the double as the organizing principle of this group;
— the bursting of the body and the emptiness;
— the lack of consistency of the object world;
— finally, the voices, the visions, the hallucinations.

It is Michelet's witch.

We shall find all these features in the women poets whom I shall introduce, and in particular Theresa, sublime Aucassine, inspired Aucassine of another time.

I have attempted to establish that woman lives under a regime of imaginary division which throws her into a reparatory narcissism. No doubt it is desirable first to explain further the content of this notion of division. Then we shall address the scopic drive which governs the female libido, in so far as woman has a narcissistic structure and pathology. From that point I shall take up the theme of female hysteria and the slave relation that woman maintains towards man, and I will conclude this chapter in the company of Theresa.

ACCESS TO THE SYMBOLIC

My thesis is that woman passes from **imaginary division** to **symbolic castration** through identification; but this identification only becomes effective to the extent that a **symbolic division** has intervened, through a properly feminine process of symbolization, starting with the mirror stage. This chronological order is completely fictitious, of course.

A certain amount of evidence is sufficient to define the female imaginary along this line of division: she has two sexual organs, dissimilar, it is true: vagina and clitoris; she is of the same sex as the parent who gives birth to her. This **double regime**, this regime of the double, becomes more specifically double on account of pregnancy and childbirth; the woman who becomes mother is no longer one, but two. From woman's point of view, she is the one who becomes double and divides into two; not the father. These data which can be called

imaginary as equally as real, were already perfectly illustrated by Anne-Marie's case. However, I insist on the fact
that women's weakness in mathematics – a weakness in which,
whether it is true or simulated, everyone indulges – finds here
its explanation and its value as a symptom.

I spoke about Philiberte in the same connection – a proper
name where I hear for myself the loss of φ – and about her
twinning fantasy which makes her spontaneously couple all
'casual' encounters, as one says. With Philiberte, we go quite
naturally from double to **loss**. I shall explain the loss of φ later
and will keep for now to **the** loss. The major event of woman's
organic life or of her physiology is surely her menstruation
or periods, also called **pertes** [loss], and, second in time,
delivery or separation (before weaning) from this part of
herself which had come imaginarily to complete her during
pregnancy, while the **pertes** had ceased, a cessation which is
the first sign of pregnancy. When she 'falls' pregnant, she no
longer 'sees' her periods. This something of herself no longer
becomes periodically visible. A woman in analysis, whom
I called Lethe, says that when her first period started, she
felt she was falling! And she actually started to fall; she was
prone to fits of vertigo of which she was only partially cured
through 'sleeping', following the advice of an aunt who had
had the same problem. Since then, she has been 'falling'
asleep unexpectedly in the middle of the day, even in her car.
She needs to take drugs to escape from sleeping. She finally
came to analysis to escape from medication. 'Falling wholly
with', such is the meaning of this transitory death.

Here is what Mary Barnes says in this connection: 'When
standing I would hold myself still and stiff, to keep together,
so as not to lose everything and go away.' For her, imaginary
division did not even intervene, or else it intervened too much
and terrified her; in any case, it is indeed only a question of
division in all the events, all the losses in the life of a woman.
They belong to various fields and could not scientifically
explain anything. But they are sufficient to circumscribe
a phenomenon of imaginary division, as a properly female
psychic regime. Woman lives with the fear of losing a part
of herself. Her husband may become this for ever lost half.
Anne-Marie has difficulty putting up with her husband's

absences, even for his work. It is worse still if he has to take a train. Inverted aggressiveness or anxiety could explain the fear of losing him. But I do not want to explain at all. The only important thing is to emphasize that she lives the least, the most legitimate absence as a final separation. 'It's absurd,' she says, 'but I can't help it.' Rather than castration anxiety, woman, as we said, knows division anxiety.

Let us restate it. The loss of a part of herself is not to be assimilated, in woman, to the fear in man of losing the penis – therefore an organ – a loss which ordinarily never happens, and loss of a quite particular organ since it is the sexual organ. It is true that the Giraffe (see chapter 2) says that if her husband abandoned her, she would feel amputated. However, she would be amputated of an organ which is not hers.

Can the term castration be used about woman? The question arises, for the very word says that the sex must take charge of this something less, this fundamental lack, otherwise one cannot speak of castration. Let us attempt to analyse further: in order for a symbolic chain to be, there needs to be a lack, which engenders demand. There is indeed for woman a real loss or waste imaginarily lived as a part of herself. But it is actually a question of a part of herself, that is to say of herself as **one**. Thus what she asks is to be given back to herself. When she comes to make love, the detumescence and the withdrawal of the penis represent quite naturally and summarize (before the future delivery) all those losses. They inscribe them retrospectively with the sign of the sex. It remains that in the sexual act, the part from which woman separates and which only covers over an ever earlier loss, has never – let us state it again – been a part of herself. She passes therefore from the real loss of an imaginary half of herself to the imaginary loss of an organ which comes to be superimposed onto these lost parts. Later, at the time of delivery, the real deprivation of a part of herself will become an imaginary frustration, through awakening the early loss of this other part of herself, her mother, from a fantasized whole. It may also become symbolic castration if it enters a symbolic chain. But how many times have we been writing this word here: **herself**?

It is because woman, **in herself**, lacks nothing, at least in the sense that she cannot come to lack any organ, except in the case of a symptomatic surgical intervention, as we said. It would actually seem that she has an extra one: the clitoris. How then does she come to consider that she is deprived of a penis? I put aside for the moment the fact that man experiences her as deprived and communicates this feeling to her, although this is not a negligible fact.

The expelling of the child and the withdrawal of the penis constitute real separations. It is the anal drive which is concerned there. As a component drive it addresses the Other from whom it expects the answer. Woman separates from something, in exchange for something else; for she asks of the Other – the man – to be taken; and as usual in this matter of gift, one no longer knows who is the beneficiary. But we recall that as a child the little girl expected a baby from the father, as a gift. It was to comfort herself from having to recognize that her mother was looking elsewhere: to the father precisely.

But then, if woman lacks nothing, what is the object of her demand? And how does she pass from imaginary division to symbolic castration? And, it could be said, how does she pass from narcissism to object libido? The transition is not obvious. 'The established idea according to which "the narcissistic libido" is the reservoir from which the "object libido" has to be extracted . . . as "a part of this libido deflected from the body proper"'; this is precisely what Jacques Lacan denounces. It is an idea which he challenges (1966). There is a 'reversing point' and not a simple cut in the same fabric. This reversing point, although it may be located in the history of the female subject at the time of the mirror stage and of childbirth, is not reducible to an historical punctuality. Woman does not pass from one structure to another; it is the **path of the drive** which is modified (Lacan, 1973).

The access to the symbolic and the 'finding of the object' are linked in one and the same process. That is how the symbolic goes hand in glove with the real.

Identification, as I said, is the process which gives woman access to symbolic castration. But that creates a problem. Woman whose fate it is to be hysterical quite naturally finds the path to identification. The only thing being that not all of

what is called identification is of the symbolic register. There
is the solicitation by the specular image; the incorporation of
the paternal phallus; finally identification properly speaking, constitutive of a possible subject, on the model of the
Fort-Da [see glossary].

Through identification with man, woman imagines she has
a penis which is lacking (whereas it is not lacking, properly
speaking, in man) and she symbolizes thus the lack of which
all the phenomena of division deprive her. She therefore passes from the imaginary loss of a half of herself to the imaginary
loss of the male sexual organ, and on to the symbolizable loss
of a sexual organ whatever it may be; provided, however,
that 'penis envy' does not fixate her to the real absence of this
particular sexual organ, the penis. But whose penis? Is the
castration which follows symbolic or only imaginary (cf. what
has been said about the Giraffe's amputation, pp. 41-2), given
that the penis has never been there in woman? Her own sexual
organ is not threatened. Another properly female process of
symbolization necessarily intervenes here, in which woman
takes herself as lost object and stake of symbolization. Losing
half of oneself in one's unity and therefore in one's being. The
symbol of lost unity is the body as a whole, without fissure.
The stake is existence itself. The specular experience is,
for the female child, a privileged moment of opening to the
symbolic play, at least when the putting together is not, on the
contrary, catastrophic.

The scopic function
To explain how the specular image may be either a symbolic
opening or a narcissistic capture, one must go back to the
scopic function.

It is this same function which organizes female libido for the
reason, no doubt, that it is also, as Lacan wrote, 'that which
eludes most perfectly the term castration'. Now, woman,
as we have said, already divided, loathes risking a new split,
that which projects the ego away: in the case in point, the
specular image [i (a)] paradoxically instructing the subject
to see itself.

For the girl, distancing is a difficult test. She prefers to
tip over into the image which (or so she believes) the equally

captive look of her mother guarantees for her, and, later, the omniscient look of the father. She, therefore, prefers believing in that image. She believes that it is herself. She merges thus with this full figure without fissure, without holes, which preserves the parental power and which is preserved by it. In doing so, she substitutes for the person of the mother who constituted the stake of the **Fort-Da**, her own person represented by her body in the specular image, image which is made to appear through the look of the mother, which she 'causes'; it is a **Fort-Da** the other way round, and it is the whole body which becomes the stake of symbolization in it, with the risks of fragmentation and hysterical paralyses which follow.

But in offering herself thus to the gaze, in showing herself, following the sequence: seeing, seeing herself, showing herself, being seen, the girl – unless she falls into the complete alienation of the hysteric – provokes the Other into an encounter and a response which gives her pleasure. Every component drive is invoking, Lacan notes. We are maybe speaking of the same thing here when we write provocation. Invocation or provocation addressed to the gaze of the Other can only intervene if the child lacks the gaze of the Same, the – fulfilling – gaze of the Mother, because this gaze precisely is occupied by the Other. It is in this play that symbolic articulation is instituted.

For henceforth the 'separation' has intervened which saves the girl from alienation. One needs to take up here another schema of Lacan's (1973):

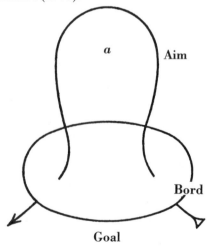

The aim and the goal that the satisfaction of the drive would be, do not coincide. If they did, the arrow would run straight. As Lacan says, the drive goes around the object (a). But it does not close on itself either; it comes back to a different point. Something has happened. This something is an incursion in the field of the Other where a response to the drive has been provoked.

This schema works as well for the scopic drive in operation from the time of the specular putting together. But, inasfar as the narcissistic resistance of woman manages to inflict the arrow of the drive to the extent of making it come back upon itself and of looping the loop, we have a phenomenon of alienating identification instead of an act of discovery of the Other (if only through the intervention of the (a)), and a scotomization of desire. What happens if the mother is fixated in the contemplation of her daughter, as of her image: for the daughter stumbles then on the bar of identification and the scopic drive comes back upon itself – missing the object (a) and the Other at the same time.

All that is left are reflections of the Same, and a hole in the place of the subject as well as of the object. If the Other of the Mother, on the contrary, functions as an interrupter, the daughter loses a luring image, but recovers her desire; and it is the Other of the Mother which becomes object of her desire. It is to the Father that she then displays herself. The onus is on this father to respond as desiring man and therefore castrated, and not as omnipotent Father-Mother gazing at himself in his creature.

If then the look of the mother turns away, the mirror breaks and the daughter repeats her experience of division, but she subsists or recovers herself as desiring object, because her mother has her own desire, which she herself cannot fulfil. Through repetition itself, the specular image with which the daughter was merged, from now on detached, and reiterating, becomes symbol of the lost unity represented by the body as one.

It is indeed the whole body which becomes here the stake of the process of symbolization, and the failure of symbolization is not expressed by any phenomena of impotence (sexual or equivalent), but by phenomena of fragmentation, or even of loss of being, or by hysterical somatizations (paralyses), localized or not.

The process is started from the moment when, operating the cut in the circuit of the scopic drive which has always governed her, the girl displays herself, instead of losing herself in the mirror. She offers herself then as object (a) and provokes the response of the Other, avoiding alienating identification. 'The incursion in the field of the Other' through provocation opens up for her then the access to the symbolic/real register. In this 'displaying' the scopic drive proper to woman makes her find her status as subject, since it is through this component drive that she demonstrates her desire of the Other and reaches it. After the encounter something has changed, since woman knows that what she wanted to see was the Other, man as subject; and that what he wanted to know was woman as point of origin, beyond the masquerade. But she cannot respond from this point of origin and he cannot respond as a subject. It is inasfar as they both accept their failure and that of the other that they have an access to the real and a gain at the symbolic level of exchange.

For man, the same thing happens, at the time of his first identification with the mother; except that, at the risk of losing his sex, he cannot be merged with her. If he denies the sex of his mother, he becomes a pervert or a fetishist; if he denies his, he becomes homosexual or impotent. The stake, here, is the sex. One can then speak of castration. For him, the specular image is less narcissistic than phallic, for it is his stature that he gains in it. The image is, as we say, orthopedic. As for the intermittent nature of the maternal gaze, it introduces him to the **Fort-Da** game, in which he identifies preferably with the Other of the mother, the Father, who has the same sex as he does, while the mother becomes the Great Other.

The girl finds all the more spontaneously the means of escaping narcissistic sleep through paternal identification, because the father meets her half way, as the abduction of Persephone shows. If her father does not desire her – does not abduct her – she is in great danger of remaining stuck to her mother. But it is true that through identifying with the Other of the mother, she runs the risk of incorporating the paternal

phallus. A passage through homosexuality, then, effectively
favours the change of object, by detaching the girl from
her mother (cf. above, p. 34). In other words, the choice of
the father cannot be lived through in panic. If the young girl
throws herself on the father, out of fear of the mother, she
will not cease throwing herself on one or the other, in fear of
being engulfed.

The master—slave couple

Woman's experience is exhausting. Deprived of an external
love object, woman wanders 'like a lost soul' and indeed turns
back to her Father: the only man who has loved her, or whom
she has been able to love. It is in him that she finds her ideal,
that is to say this unity that she lacks since she is divided.
And when she loves another man, she loves him as she loved
her father. She makes a Father out of him, a Father-mother
actually. She wants him to desire her and to give her life. She
expects everything from him. Her whole demand is located in
what I call 'the prosopopoeia of Femininity', and it is hardly
ironical, for it is true that women walk in the street or stay at
home like allegories, and that they speak all the same.

Thus, Femininity speaks and she says:

*I am weak; the slightest thing ruffles me. I am gift made
woman. I don't belong to myself. Without you I am nothing.
I expect everything from you. Please do not go away. When
you're not here, I don't exist. I shall be as you want, beautiful,
childlike, but passionate as well. I shall be your mistress,
your wife, your sister and your mother, all in one, and even
your friend. But on the* **condition** *that you love me.*

This prosopopoeia, as we see, contains a deal. Woman gives
herself totally in exchange for love.

For she is entirely suspended to the desire of the Other, as
long as she has not discovered her own desire. And there is
no other way for her of discovering her own desire than to go
through the desire of the Other. ('Woman is alterocentric,'
Gina Lombroso was already saying in 1924, in *L'âme de la
femme*). It is probably what has been called her passivity.
A passivity which orders her to know the penis, although she
does not admit that that is what she is looking for, because

in fact she does not know. She continues to deny her genital drive, and sometimes her pleasure. She thus remains dependent, without her own declared desire: in one word slave of a master whom she gives to herself and who agrees to enter this relationship which appears to him, wrongly as we shall see, advantageous. The terms of this relationship are the following, and it is the woman who poses them: if you leave me, I die. We have seen with what permanence these two terms, separation and death mark, designate, draw the line of imaginary division of woman and occupy her libidinal field. As in all master-slave relations of this kind, there is of course alienation and a certain loss of something from the start: for either you leave me and I die; or you don't leave me and I lose myself, since I become you. In any case I do not live. Same false alternative as that of freedom or life, for either I lose life, or I lose freedom and the freedom of living (Lacan, 1973). It seems that man would rather say: 'If you leave me, I'll kill you.' It is, at least, what Mariella Righini says in a survey on suicide, to oppose this male attitude to that of woman who says: 'If you leave me, I'll kill myself' (Righini, 1975).

So, woman makes herself the slave of man, in exchange for a little love. In doing so, she loses her life, if not life. She is this subject who, as any subject, only takes meaning in the field of the Other (man or child) and vanishes at the same time as subject. She is invocating in relation to the Other; she is invocation itself and that is why she may be taken as the origin of language, as Dante's Beatrice. But she spontaneously alienates herself according to the mode of coupling of the master and the slave. She has always been installed in the alternative: life or death. It is the lethal Lacanian vel [Latin for 'or' – used in logic as proposing no alternative]: either she installs herself in the death of Narcissus; or she gets herself recognized by the Other and loses herself as subject, because she identifies with the desire of the Other.

However the master-slave couple, like the man-woman couple, is to be taken as a couple, as a relation; and not as two terms both positively marked; otherwise one posits two races and the 'old dream of symmetry', denounced by Luce Irigaray, takes shape again. The solution is not in the refusal of this relation; it is not in denial.

'Through which the subject finds the path of return from the vel of alienation, which was called the other day separation,' wrote Lacan (1973). Separation, second moment of repetition of which the first is alienation – saves from alienation. But to separate is precisely 'to adorn oneself [se parer] with the Other'. The return path is narrow. The whole difficulty for woman, as for any slave, lies there: being the cut, how could she afford the luxury, moreover, of cutting herself from the other herself? The fate of the master, as we know, is not any happier. If the slave-woman loses her freedom and chooses to live, if only as a loser, man keeps his identity and his name which he transmits, in our society at least; but he is often no more than a name.

The time of separation is not easy to pinpoint. It is a question for the woman of not identifying with the Other. But to enjoy him – in order to enjoy him. This time comes when she admits that she only enjoys the Signifier – as such, representing a subject for another signifier which represents it. For woman enjoys this: the very revelation of the Other as signifier. She enjoys the phallus (and not solely the penis; the Giraffe who would feel amputated if she was abandoned, confesses at the same time that she has become 'sexually indifferent', and yet she is not a frigid woman) as the one who puts her in place, as barred subject, gives her thus access to symbolic castration (which symbolic division had made possible since she was already posited in it as separate).

We have said that with the child she passes from 1 to 2 and even 3, including the father. But there, too, she personally needs to separate from the imaginary other as part of herself, in order to recognize the Other as signifier, as one. Her problematic is indeed that which makes her pass from half to double, then from double to 1, 2, 3, etc. She acquires this simple calculation with difficulty, because what she lives in her being is rather a 'trampling down'. If she only becomes 1 through the other, which makes 2, her unity as subject is always precarious. She risks crushing into zero. And if she only becomes 1 through the fact of the Other, whose signifier is the phallus, she can only be a phallus – not identical to the second one, certainly (or rather to the first one); but then what is she?

No doubt one cannot desire what is lacking. The **wanting what is needed** would be closer to what moves woman (eternally unsatisfied, as they say), with the inflexion that the closeness of will communicates to wanting; and with needing rather than lacking, because she needs at each new step.

To save their relation, man, on the other hand, attempts to identify with woman. But he then goes against his vocation. It is, as we have said, the sex change which compensates for the failure of exchange. If man can identify with woman, it is quite evidently because the process of identification finds a support in him as well, in his own organization. This support is the foreskin, which is, as Amado Levy-Valensi says 'formally woman because the penis moves in it'. Whatever his organs are, he has also made a primary identification with the mother.

Circumcision and other rituals may make man more virile. But he remains capable of identification. We have been able to establish a kind of sexual equivalence between male sexual act and delivery; I quoted Ferenczi in that connection. But whoever says sex change, reciprocal identification, says failure of exchange, since, at best, one becomes the other, one misses and annihilates the other. It is the deadlock of unisex. The pernicious dream of the hippies for which women have already found a remedy. Marguerite Duras and Xavière Gauthier tell us in *Les parleuses* (Duras and Gauthier, 1974) that some women deliberately gather away from men in hermetic communities 'to find themselves'. These communities of women recall the 'provençal rooms' where men used to gather in the last century away from women who were forbidden entry to these circles, 'even to do the housework'. The ethnologist who applied himself to find the reason for it did not find any other than the very severity of this single rule and its effects (Roubin, 1970). In fact, women on one side, men on the other, segregate themselves to escape the ever threatening and repeated contamination.

To come back to woman, she quite likes to play the man, but as for prestige, that she leaves to him, she used to leave to him. . . She is left with, as we saw, the return path after separation, or sublimation of her love. Seeing that man escapes her, for he does not willingly settle in identification and rushes after an other salvaging (a) (in order not to be castrated); after having made him impotent precisely through forbidding him objects (a), causes of his desire, she shouts her love to him; then she writes it to herself in her so-called intimate diaries; then she writes it.

Writing love is the solution of sublimation, the one which saves woman from nymphomania and erotomania. We are not concerned here with the natural path, where, wife and mother, she finds a way of blossoming: it is a more difficult path to locate and extricate. But we do not deny it; we think that it takes its entire meaning from the extreme paths represented by pathology on the one hand and sublimation on the other.

THERESA

We come to Theresa who made God speak. I shall not deal with the mystical Theresa, but only with the woman she was. As far as the whole of her mystical experience is concerned, I take her word, since I have not had that experience. Therefore I believe that what she says is true from the outset; it is true since she says it: 'In the intimate union with God, all she can do is enjoy.' That is what she says. And I believe that she enjoys.

I do not think that one can say that Theresa's love object is hallucinated. Her experience unfolds in the real, despite imaginary errings. The question for her is precisely to recover from her pathological excesses, from her numerous hysterical pains (that is the word she uses herself) through the exercises of a mystical experience. And everything lies there: from her knowing that the sexual relation fails since there is only jouissance from the word spoken to the real other, Theresa was able to elaborate her mystic.

If I come to speak of Theresa at this point in my argument, it is because she has loved, essentially; and as a woman, inasmuch as she spoke her love. She even wrote it, like Sappho, like Louise Labé. The distance is less from Theresa to Louise Labé – who both only loved men – than from Sappho to Theresa; for Sappho only loved her mother and her daughter to whom she gave her mother's name: Kleis. What better proof could she give of an equal love? The same goes for

Madame de Sévigné or Colette. Now, 'the affective incest with the mother,' as Dr Wolff points out (1971), 'is the essential of sapphism'.

There is another woman, both poet and in love: the one whom Pierre de Mandiargues resurrected, Isabelle Mora. Poet, she loved a poet whom she had never met; and she was loved by him in such a perfect way that a meeting would not have added anything to that love, for it was entirely consumed in poetry. But mainly, no force in the world could put an obstacle to it; not even that of jealous and brutal brothers. Tahar Labib Djedidi (1974), describing a process of 'sexualization of the Arab language', quotes some exemplary cases of spoken love: 'Numerous are the tales where a lady from a good family lets herself be seduced or almost seduced, not by the poet, but by his poetry. The word alone is able to unveil the lady.'

Just as exemplary is the case of Aimée (Lacan, 1973). Aimée was sending a sonnet each week to the Prince of Wales. He did not reply; for Aimée, the machine to speak love was broken down. But failed or not, it was love spoken and lived poetically; like the love of Ulrich and his sister Agatha in *The Man without Qualities* (Musil, 1930), although in this latter case the incest was consummated! Even though it cannot be certain, so evasive is the text. Ulrich and Agatha are only carried away in the irresistible union of their bodies to the extent that they first unite in words. 'Love is essentially loquacity', declares Musil-Ulrich. To say that love is lived through the word, is to say that it is not lived at the level of the sexes, and we are back with Theresa.

Theresa, then, loved her father and was loved by her father (whereas the empress in *Die Frau ohne Schatten*, we may recall, rose against her father – God – and said no to him). It is her mother who brought Theresa down. If one reads between the lines, one notes that the only person whom Theresa reproaches in some way (considering politeness), is her mother, and for having communicated to her the taste for tales of chivalry. A curious reproach, since she has thus taught love to her. So Theresa loves her father; she also loves one of her brothers with whom she used to play, as a child, at building monasteries; she loves her confessors, and she loves

St John of the Cross, Father Gratian and Joseph, 'much
more helpful to mortals than the queen of angels', because he
was the father of God on earth, a father therefore. She is a
hommosexual, following the Lacanian spelling; and it is as a
man that she is going to found an order. We shall, however,
see which one. The same goes for George Sand: undertaking
to write her autobiography, she forgets herself and tells her
father's life: this Napoleonic hero, her ideal lover. To the
extent that publishers and readers protest. Theresa, like
George Sand, like any woman writer, can only at first pass
through a male identification; Marguerite Duras, too, speaks
of this inevitable 'aping'.

Goethe in *Elective Affinities* (see above, pp. 21-2) tells
how the naive Edward started to love Odile (while he adored
his wife Charlotte) when he discovered that she had taken on
the same writing as himself: 'He looked at Odile and again
at the papers: the end in particular was absolutely as if he
had written it himself. Odile was silent, but was looking in
his eyes with the strongest joy. Edward raised his arms: you
love me Odile, you love me!' And consequently he loved her.
Goethean men are thus made, and others. But can Odile,
beyond the first moment of love, renounce her own writing?
As for Edward, Goethe admits, if he kisses and kisses again
the beginning of the document, 'he hardly dares kiss the end,
because he thinks he is seeing his own writing'(!).

The refusal, if not the repression, of her own sexuality cost
Theresa dearly, since her decision to enter religion after the
death of her mother resulted in an illness of several years.
The violence of her somatic conversion expresses the violence
of her repressed desire. She very nearly dies, and cannot
swallow anything (I emphasize, for the oral theme will come
back in force on another occasion): fever, pains in the heart
and fainting, vomiting, etc. She remains paralysed for three
or four years, and will have to learn to walk again on all fours,
an example which illustrates well, it seems to me, what I was
saying earlier: the body becomes symbol of the lost unity and,
as such, it is it which speaks in phenomena of somatization.
In this case, it becomes impotent, in the same way as man's
penis may be unable to move.

From her father, Theresa goes on to God, but not without

ensuring that she paves the way in the person of the fathers who confess her and guarantee her actions and her words for her.

It is all she asks from men anyway: to be fathers. No mention is made of the penis. It will return sublimated, in the shape of the wafer. And Theresa says ingenuously that she liked them very big.

St John of the Cross, aware of her greed, broke one into pieces one day when he was giving her communion. Theresa made the best of it, since she had decided to accept everything, but experienced nonetheless a persisting vexation. It is quite true that this voracity betrays an identificatory oral function strongly operating in her. Similarly, the supreme expression of her love is oral. 'O that you would kiss me with the kisses of your mouth!', as it is said in the Song of Songs (I, 2).

She does not lack the knowledge that if she identifies with God, she commits a sin of pride; and even that calling herself his beloved daughter or his wife could be of devilish inspiration. That is why she dismisses any desire of her own, any will of her own, and leaves it up to father X or Y to know if her vision is vision or not and if the word of God is the word of God. It is what the author Marcelle Auclair calls 'her angelic ruses'. She cannot really go as far as gobbling up God, only to remain with nothing or nobody in front of her at the end, which is the fate of all hysterics.

Theresa is no more shrewd than humble. She has made humility into the main and unique tool of the mystical practice: if she is nothing, God is all, as long as she is nothing, as far as God wants it, and always a bit less in order not to have her own being or will.

Humility, if we want to keep this term, is the peg of her entire experience. At each step towards a superior mystical state, Theresa fortifies herself with humility. Thus she avoids anything that could today be considered feminine grievance. She does not want to be the equal of men. With men lie power, titles, decision-making, judgment and competence. 'In every man there is a marine' echoes Marguerite Duras. Women have no need to deal with all these 'subtleties' which charm men, Theresa notes. It is true that men have from birth a toy at their disposal.

She, therefore, knows that she looks after her soul in loving God; that she has no other path to recover herself as subject; because if the Great Other is, he is **one** in relation to her, and with her, it makes at least two. She therefore is also **one**.

Thus she goes from the double which she had nevertheless liked during her coquettish adolescence as a pretty woman, to the **one**, and she exists for the length of time it takes her to recognize it. But in order not to identify with God, to enjoy God – and there is no doubt that she enjoys him – in this extreme peril of annihilation, humility is no longer enough. The separation from God is the making of a **third party** who guarantees it, in the event her confessors. She needs to be assured that it is God who speaks to her. 'It is true that in a certain way making love takes three people', Marguerite Duras writes.

The existence of this Other, the Lord whom she enjoys, is only guaranteed by a third who operates the cut, who intervenes to say it: 'Yes, it is God who speaks to you and to whom you speak, you are two.' At that point, she can move far enough away from God to know that she enjoys and can remain 'active', they are her own words. It is the opposite of the kiss with merged mouths of Aucassine and of the single mouth of Freud. Thus woman needs a third to know that with the Other it made two. Maybe we are giving here the entirely abstract schema of an intervention in the analysis of a woman. (It is this third which is lacking in the feminine world of Aucassine; apart from that, everything is there: mysticism, voices, visions, love and poetry.)

If there is no other word than the word spoken to the Other, Theresa speaks. And more generally woman, governed as she is by the invocating drive. That is how woman is at the origin of language, at the origin of human society, at the location of passage, of separation, at the cut; she is this cut. But she doesn't know it. She needs man to tell her; otherwise she forgets herself as one. And then 1 + 1 no longer make 2, and the whole male social edifice collapses. Woman undermines male constructs. More directly, she castrates man through refusing his penis, in favour of the phallus – father-God. She castrates him as radically through loving his penis only, at the expense of the man.

Thus she castrates man right up to the sexual act. She castrates him still through understanding nothing in what he does. Theresa says,

Beware of using and tiring your thoughts in this research. Women need nothing that goes beyond their understanding. It is a favour that God will do us when His majesty wishes it and we will discover that we have learnt everything without care or work . . . I therefore strongly recommend, when you are listening to a sermon or meditating the mysteries of our Holy Faith, that you do not tire or use your thoughts in looking for subtleties; it is not for women; and many of these things are not even for men.

It is in this last remark that one measures the signification of this refusal to understand, which she strongly reiterates in her commentary on the Song of Songs – written at the instruction of Father Gratian – and also in this fundamental statement: '**I say it to women and men, they do not have to sustain truth with their science**' (my emphasis).

Women's fortune today is that success, science and power are discredited. Make way for the slaves! Let us hope that women will think before claiming victory.

The only knowledge is revealed through the **jouissance** of the love of the Other. That knowledge is the privilege of women. It makes men's science obsolete. If men were not forced to love, they would no longer be poet; they would no longer invent their language. In their annihilating rage of naming everything, already denounced by Jean Genet (a man, it is true, but homosexual) in *The Balcony* (1962), they would lose language itself. What happens is always a bit like this. Language has a disease, we could say nowadays, as we say of trees or cattle. It proliferates.

It is true that when woman does not love, nothing is forbidden to her any longer. And that when she loves, everything is allowed to her. Love is thus the most active of the solvents of institutions. But through that very fact, being nobody, and to that extent eluding any authority, woman for ever has to invent a new language.

To summarize . . .

Here is woman as we have described her: for ever divided, for ever deprived of half of herself, narcissistically divided between subject and object, in any case an orphan. In one word, narcissist by structure and fated to division.

And we repeat our question: how does she go from imaginary division to symbolic castration which controls the entry into language?

Through a process of **identification**, of which the first terms have been solicitation by [i (a)], then incorporation of the ego ideal, namely the phallus, then identification with the desire of the Other, and finally, after separation or cut, love. Such are the four stages of the shaping of the subject in woman, at the end (in any case hypothetical) of which she speaks. But at the time of contamination through man of the fear of losing the penis (which for her becomes the feeling of never having had it), it cannot be said that there is truly symbolic castration in woman. There is superimposition of male castration onto female imaginary division, substitution of one fear for another. There is then a castration which is only imaginary. It becomes symbolic when it is grafted onto the symbolic division which has already intervened.

Identification proper is the one which is at work in the game of **Fort-Da** where the characters slide on top of one another like cards. The subject can then say: I cut, and in its cut, be instituted, so that it is then affirmed in the very sliding of the cards. It is the cut which makes the way out of alienation possible. We saw that it is not necessary to wait, other than in a fictitious becoming; for the cut possibly intervenes from the time of the specular image.

Woman's weakness is the result of this vocation for identification which makes her a stranger to herself, and of this mitigated status. As a subject, she is easily displaced and develops a permanent imaginary agency which protects her from disintegration, dividing into two and loss of being.

But she also gains an advantage from the very fact that she is a slave, subjected rather than subject; and from the fact that she has been despised: she is left indeed with **jouissance**. And it is to the very extent that she enjoys that she is silent. There are no words to tell **jouissance**. But only words of love which tell and do not tell. It is the major contradiction experienced by all women writers and by the exemplary Theresa.

And yet she is indeed at the origin of human language, in that she 'procures' children for man, that is to say in that she makes the generation which is constituent of social organization possible; and in that she invents the speech of love, that which invokes the Other. She is thereby in the symbolic from the start; but she repetitively falls into the imaginary.

On top of inventing the speech of love, woman has the gift for pythic speech, as we shall see later in connection with a heroine of Goethe, the astrologist Macarie. She therefore has several language modes at her disposal: the prosopopoeia of femininity; the pastiche of the hommosexual; pythic speech; and the speech of love. The unconscious speaks for the one who listens in any of these four modes, pythic language not being privileged at all in its relation to the unconscious, for it is still a knowledge which does not know itself. Thus woman can be analysand and analyst in the same way as man.

Besides, does the unconscious have a sex?

It is possible to locate in this very text the layers of these four modes of female speaking and moreover to hear the unconscious in it.

4

Brother and sister

I know that you are a woman beautiful to
behold; and when the Egyptians see you,
they will say, 'This is his wife'; then they
will kill me, but they will let you live.
Say you are my sister . . .

Genesis XII, 11-13

— Olivier Guichard, what are women for
a politician?
— Myself, I only had a sister. To have a
sister is to have the experience of a couple
very early; you protect her intensely and
you shudder at her follies.

Extract from *Cris et Chuchotements*, by
Gonzagues Saint-Bris, in *Elle*, 31 March 1975

IF there is a spoken love it is, on the one hand, indeed brother-and-sister love, a love which appears entirely natural; and, on the other, the analytic model, since the analytic relation is the counterpart of the sexual relation, at least inasfar as intervention functions in it like the manifestation of an other desire against which demand stumbles; the index of an other subject; it being understood that the aim there is quite other.

The model of brotherly relation is given by Musil in *The Man without Qualities* (Luccioni, G., 1959). Ulrich and his sister Agatha, male and female emanations of one and the same being which is remarkable and singular in every aspect, begin again the tale of the perfect **fraternal couple** related a hundred times in German literature: that of Thomas Mann amongst others. Here is what Michel Tournier — as it happens — says about the Mann family in his preface to *Mephisto* (1981):

Be it, for example, the theme of fraternal incest which keeps
haunting Thomas Mann who takes it up in 1905 in his short

story Wälsungenblut *['The blood of the Walsungs'] and deals with it at length in his novel* The Holy Sinner *(1951). Nothing in the life of the author seems to connect with it. However, his wife Katia Mann had a twin brother called Klaus whom – if we can tell from the photos at our disposal – his nephew strikingly resembled. The couple Katia-Klaus was so notoriously inseparable that the publication of* Wälsungen-blut *created a scandal and the issues of the magazine* Neue Rundschau *where the short story had been published had to be withdrawn.*

The publication, since then, of *Gemini* (1975) throws some light on this insistence of Tournier's in speaking about brotherly incest. It is the story of two twin brothers. Michel Tournier himself said about this novel, in a radio interview in August 1975, that twins make 'the ideal couple, sterile and eternal; other couples are only satellites of it; they live in vicissitudes'. *Gemini* in turn throws light on *Friday or the Other Island* with which I shall deal in the next chapter in connection with hermaphroditism: it is remarkable after all that Robinson, the man alone, has lost a young sister whose memory haunts him.

Tournier, even though he knows Germany well, as *The Erl-King* testifies, is not German; nor are Pascal, Chateaubriand, Renan and so many others. But it is true that one finds in German literature the persisting trace of the myth of twins. And then there is Goethe and his sister, Nietzsche and his sister, etc. Is it surprising if the 'et ta soeur?' [used like the English 'go fuck yourself'; lit. 'what about your sister?'] of vulgar belligerence comes out with no apparent reason, to evoke the embarrassing and hidden thing.

The embarrassing and hidden thing in the brother-and-sister relation, is the sex of the sister and even her vulva. For the Mashona and the Matabele of Africa, 'the word **totem** also means **my sister's vulva**', reports Myriam Pécaut (1974-5) in connection with the equivalence incest/cannibalism and food. And she adds: 'It would seem that the incestuous object here is firstly the sister.'

The model of this relation, as we said, because in it it is accepted up to its extreme and fatal consequence, is that of

Ulrich and Agatha in *The Man without Qualities*. When Ulrich sees his sister, he fancies her. 'She is a tall thin Pierrot, with a **dry**, scented skin' (my emphasis) (whereas Diotimes has small chubby hands), with small breasts and long slender limbs. She is the female double of Ulrich. 'A hermaphrodite', he thinks. 'The human being comes in two shapes, man and woman.' But these shapes are secondary, unreal in some way, and in order to find the lost unity, alive and true, they have to be added to each other. 'It would seem that brother and sister have already gone half way' towards the lost unity to be found.

With Agatha, everything is possible because she will really do anything. She is the only character in this novel who is free, unconstructed. The mad Clarissa is unconstructed but quite mad; the Arheims and Diotimes are falsely constructed; Ulrich himself is deconstructed and 'without qualities', but out of a willing refusal of the everyday, the social, history and even incarnation. Agatha herself is a miracle of true spontaneity. She is authentic, outside of any structure, an outlaw. Perfectly 'vacant' but without suffering, as opposed to the rebellious Ulrich. She does not seek. She waits. She **sleeps** (the emphasis is mine) as much as possible while waiting. When passion comes, it will take all of her.

For Ulrich, she is the link with mystical life, with communion beyond the world, in defiance of this Cacanie (Austro-Hungarian empire) which is the very image of the human community mummified in its categories, its historical and geographical forms. The Great War will explode this whole high society. Crime alone is an answer to inanity. Through lack of finding the living unity, beyond the ossifying layers of reason, man turns hatefully against man; and in crime, at least, can breathe normally again.

There is – as another solution – the mystical Agatha. It is clear that this love, at first spoken throughout a period of 'sacred conversations', then consummated, or nearly so, is also a crime. Not for moral reasons. But because it is an attack on creation, a refusal of birth, the μή φῦναι so forcefully picked up by Lacan in his seminar on *Ethics* (1960) but which drifts [**dérive**] 'on the desire for a good' [**bien**; both 'good' and 'goods']: the nostalgic good of the parental union: 'Love between brother and sister', says Kafka, more or less, in a letter to his sister Valli taken up by Musil, 'is repetition of the love of the father and mother'.

It is a question of denying the accident of birth proper and the 'secondary' separate states which follow, in order to find again the unity of being. Musil takes it out on existence because it does not exist enough.

Ulrich and Agatha may consummate their love (which would not happen in Goethe) in a paroxysm of passion which finds its only duplication, at least if it really is consummated, in the final scene of *The Mother* by Bataille (1966); and for a good reason, because in both cases it is a question of incest. After which there is only death.

Agatha, who ignores good and evil, commits suicide. Mystical spoken love was not possible because (this is my emphasis) of the bodies. Neither was consummated love, because ecstasy does not last. Thus Musil demonstrates that one can reach real life, but not live it. Ulrich goes to war (that of 1914). One can bet that he will behave as a hero. It is a male solution which makes up for the accident of birth through a willingly incurred risk. Clarissa becomes (was) mad. It is an epilogue of woman. The other characters, who were moral and had ideals, will certainly continue – if war allows it – to serve them. They will live for truth, if not in truth; and thus they will be occupied.

It is only in appearance that Musil's fraternal couple contradicts the wholly platonic couple dreamed of by Goethe. I deliberately leave aside the dull play *Die Geschwister* (1776) ['Brothers and sisters']. It is more similar to the bourgeois and tearful dramas of the French eighteenth century than to a romantic drama; moreover, as far as we are concerned, the title alone is to be retained: it is not in this play that we shall find the model of the Goethean brotherly couple, since there is a misunderstanding about the kinship link announced in the title – which does not take its signification away.

Rather we shall trace this couple everywhere else in Goethe's voluminous works; in each of his sentences, in practically each of his words; for one can find in them a veiled reference to his own couple, the one he formed with his sister Cornelia. He says himself in his autobiography (*Goethes*

Werke) that she was only one and a half years younger than
he, and that circumstances had strongly bonded them together: 'Returning from these excursions undertaken half for
pleasure, half with an artistic intention . . . I was pulled
back home by a truly magnetic force which had always very
strongly acted upon me: it was my sister.' The severity and
the age of the father seem to have added even more to these
'circumstances'. The brother and the sister were closer to
their relatively young and lively mother. It is consequently a
position of withdrawal which both had adopted in view of an
ever threatening paternal confrontation.

'We thought ourselves very unhappy and indeed we were,'
Goethe writes, 'since blood ties prevented us from converting
our position of confidants into that of lovers.' One could not
be clearer. And it is even possible to add: so they had thought
of it?

Death snatched this beloved sister away from Goethe; he
then conceived the project of bringing her back to life in
a poetic work. A project which was unrealized and no doubt
unrealizable. But if he was not able to make of his sister the
deliberate object of a particular piece of work, on the other
hand his whole work, both overall and in detail, is the shadow
of the 'wonderful soul' and its 'magical mirror' at the same
time.

Thus all the novels and plays of Goethe reproduce the same
scenario: the brother and the sister live together with a child
of one **or** the other whom they raise and whose other real
parent is dead. In *Wilhelm Meister's Years of Travel* (1829a)
M. de Brevanne lives in a castle with his sister and her son.
The whole tale is placed under the sign of Joseph and of **the
flight into Egypt.** Lothario believes he has discovered that
he is Charlotte's brother, because he has been her mother's
lover, and he renounces Charlotte. In *The Man of Fifty*, the
Major lives with his sister, the Baroness and her daughter,
Hilary. 'From the time of her youth, the Baroness has loved
her brother to the extent of preferring him to all men, and
perhaps Hilary's inclination (for her uncle) has been, if not
provoked, at least surely maintained by this preference.'

(In connection with which the declaration of a woman
analysand irresistibly comes back to me like an echo; on the

eve of her wedding, some thirty years earlier, she had written
to her brother: 'In any case, I shall never love a man as much
as you.')

When one reads, afterwards, the short play mentioned
above, *Die Geschwister*, and one hears Marianne making
her fervent declarations to her 'brother', Goethe tells us
afterwards in vain that she is only the daughter of Charlotte,
whom William once loved (yet another Charlotte: yet another
defunct love!), and not his own sister; for we are not persuaded. It is indeed a disavowed brotherly passion which is
in question.

In any case, the couple retains something incestuous, which
characterizes all Goethean couples, since, in defiance of generations, the lover or the mistress always loves the daughter
or the son of their partner.

There is a major obstacle there, postulated from the start,
and which takes on its full meaning from the fact that it is
often gratuitous. There isn't the shadow of any real obstacle
to the union of Werther and Charlotte, since she is not even
officially engaged to Albert at the time of their first meeting.
Yet both postulate that they are for ever divided: 'Ah! If she
could have turned him into a brother at that moment! How
happy she would have been if she could have married him to
one of her friends!'

The 'Say you are my sister' of the unglorious declaration
of Abraham, written as an epigraph to this chapter, could
jokingly serve as epigraph to the whole of Goethe's work. The
major obstacle, from the start to the consummation of the
couple, is not put there solely to make the good people cry.
Later Goethe will turn it into a maxim for living: 'The state of
fiancé is the most pleasant that is granted us in civilized life',
he has the blessed Macarie say (*Maximen und Reflexionen*,
1907).

Wilhelm Meister's Years of Travel has as a subtitle *The
Renunciants* and we know that Wilhelm and Nathalie have
imposed 'prescriptions' on themselves which recall the code
of courtly love. He has to leave on a trip, he must not return
before a year and must not spend more than three days under
the same roof. It is a test. But also a way for both to live
their love in chastity. Goethe writes to Eckermann: 'Opposed

felicity, **hindered** action, **unsatisfied** desires are not **handi-
caps** particular to a period, but those of all men. And it
would be a shame if, at least once in their life, everyone did
not go through a period of time when Werther would seem to
have been written for them' (original emphasis). One could
not better describe castration as human condition. The important thing for us present-day readers is not that Charlotte
is Albert's fiancée, but that Werther can speak thus: 'She is
sacred for me. All desire **quietens in her presence.**' And at
the highest moment of his passion, 'it is like a wall of **separation** which rose before my soul'. And, shortly before dying,
he writes still: 'Is not the love I have for her the **healthiest,**
the **purest**, the most **brotherly** love?' Such is Goethe's ideal:
a brotherly love. Thus he will marry a woman whom he will
not be able to love, because she is in no way a sister, another
himself; but on the contrary, so foreign that he has nothing to
say to her. And the legitimate son whom he will have by her will
remain far from his heart, behind the illegitimate children,
or the orphans, whose education he enjoys organizing in his
writings.

At the time of Werther, he has not yet rationalized his
favourite motif by making sexual abstinence the essential
principle of the practice of *The Renunciants*; he does not yet
know that the rule of abstinence has no other (conscious) aim
than the survival of desire. Later he will write: 'When I am
in desire, I seek pleasure, and when I have pleasure, I regret
desire.' Renunciation is therefore the main consideration.
It is, then, for Goethe a question of reaching an optimum of
pleasure. Man is limited. It is **his condition.** As opposed to
Musil's *The Man without Qualities* who refuses any deter-
mination, the Goethean man accepts his limits, we would say
castration.

The society of La Tour has more to do with courses on
love than with a spiritual community. Goethe remains, deep
down, opposed to marriage and procreation. Or rather he
will separate these two functions; there will be his 'Lady', and
on the other hand, his wife. It is because his Renunciants are
marked by repressed, unrecognized brotherly passion. Their
ethics are only secondarily the fruit of a truly free wisdom.
Goethe oscillates between what Lacan calls 'the service of

the good', in the event, for him, calculated renunciation, interested chastity; and on the other hand (on the contrary) the discovery of absolute desire in the beyond of good. Thus, as opposed as the wise Goethe is to Musil's Ulrich (he is even more so to the hard and pure Agatha) he is nevertheless, like him and like the troubadours, asocial.

No doubt it can be said that the primary model of courtly love is this brotherly love, beause of the sterility of the couple and its chastity, and also the valorization of the woman perversely offered to the contemplation of the impotent man. This is the manner (minus sexuality) in which Hegel describes it:

The relation in its unmixed form is found, however, in that between brother and sister. They are the same blood which has, however, in them reached a state of rest and equilibrium. Therefore, they do not desire one another, nor have they given to, or received from, one another this independent being-for-self; they are free individualities in regard to each other. (Hegel, 1905, p. 274)

That there is **no desire** is more than problematic. But it is true that neither of them knows that they have a desire, if they are about the same age.

Things will get complicated if one of them is half way between two generations. It is the case of the woman analysand whose letter I have mentioned and whom I shall call by a man's name, Procustes, which sounds female to me. Her brother is twelve years older than she. Their father died when she was fifteen and her brother twenty-seven. He replaced his father at the head of a very large family business and has not stopped privileging his sister at the expense of an older sister, denied by **both**. However, there has not been any question of desire between them. Which does not prevent Procustes from writing to her brother who has remained single, on the eve of her marriage, the definitive words which I quoted and which are exactly what the Baroness said to her brother, in Goethe. For Procustes these words came true. She knew a lot of men. But all things considered . . . they never measured up to her brother. At the death of the yardstick-brother, and after so many failures, she became so depressed that she could only recognize the truth of this old naive declaration which took on the value of fate.

But the characteristic of brother and sister is to belong to the same **generation**. That everything gets muddled and complicated when the age difference increases, only serves to indicate better what is the natural inclination of this kind of love: the sister then seizes the opportunity of putting her brother in the place of her father. The fact remains that if they are children contemporarily, they contemporarily go through their latency period and one does not know before the other that he desires the other; moreover, neither are they able to know that they desire **elsewhere**, as is the case in the mother/son or father/daughter couples (not to mention homosexual combinations which are just as virulent). Quite sheltered behind this ignorance, they can surrender to their love, so they believe, without danger. We know that childish erotic games and pubertal awakenings are not without attempts at seduction. But both the brother and the sister remain nevertheless persuaded of the sacred and pure nature of their relation – their innocence being on a par with their relative sexual impotence. They remain therefore a child for each other and, as such, in some way, **sacred**.

If the adelphic* Oedipus prevails following the real death of the father, for example (as is the case for Procustes), neither can get free from him, precisely because neither is adult enough to desire elsewhere (as the father desires the mother) at the time when the youngest seeks him as lover in the platonic meaning of the word. Consequently at no time is there any resolution of the Oedipus whose adelphic link is avoidance.

The brother and the sister order sex through their sole **opposition**, from their postulated **resemblance** (same origin), by scotomizing a more fundamental **difference**. Besides, it is not true that they have the same origin. Born at different times, they are born of different parents. But they want their parents, like essences, to be immutable. They already deny the contingency of their respective birth. 'We are twins', exclaims Agatha despite the five years between her and Ulrich. From this postulated native equation, they develop a system

---

* That is to say, peculiar to brothers.

of secondary oppositions and resemblances where sexual difference and desire are spirited away. It is not true that blood is there in equilibrium and at rest. There is only denial of sexuality and ideal love: the brother being, in our society, the holder of genius; and the sister of beauty. A way of saying: **brother/sister, he/she [le/la] which would not be sexual.** The masculine and the feminine in a pure state, in itself, we could say. We may wonder how such a process presents itself in a country like Hungary, where the language does not allow for the translation of a title like 'Her and him'.

Thus the natural difference of the sexes becomes ethical in the brother-and-sister couple, if one wishes to take up Hegel's terms and his analysis: not because the natural relation between the members of a family is ethical, any more than are the singular relations of each of them, and the sexual relation less so than any other; but because, on the contrary, any sublimated relation is ethical.

Already, indeed, as he/she, as beauty and genius, the brother and the sister each quite naturally find their 'actuality' in themselves. They have no need to make a child – or so they believe. Genius destines the brother to his life in the world, and beauty destines the sister to eternally being the phallus of the brother and keeper of his phallus. One way of dedicating oneself to death. Antigone is for ever. It is a religious marriage which ties her to her brother; mystical even, as Musil saw clearly. In a way, this union denies the family (to come) and society itself. There lies its contradiction. But how could any brotherly couple not fall into the trap? The unconscious is scotomized there from the start; the couple settles in the symbolic-religious order, peacefully, for life, without guessing that one day the unconscious will present the bill. What a saving, if it were possible!

Thus this couple speaks. They both have the same language and more exactly the same signifiers. Or so they believe. But there lies their fatal illusion: this perfect understanding on which Goethe, Thomas Mann and Musil insist, so perfect (and how is it that they have not noticed the crack?) that they no longer even have to speak, what is it made of? No longer any need to speak indeed. But since it is a question of a spoken love, on what is this love going to subsist?

Whatever their words, they do not make love, even if once they played at making it. I am not concerned here with the very different cases when they went on for years. I posit that the characteristic of this relation is abstinence and that if they did play during their childhood, they forgot it in a hurry.

Those chose to be the other, instead of having the other, like Goethe and Cornelia, following the law of identification recalled earlier (Lemoine, G. and P. (1972), and cf. above, p. 33). The most masculine, at the end of the process of identification, is not the one we think; it is always the other, as in marriage in any case. Antigone becomes the family hero, and Procustes deserves her male Christian name at last. 'My Lord', such is the title that the knight gives his revered suzerain Lady, through a reversal, quite chivalrous of course, of the relation (Maillet, 1975). But then what does the knight become? A troubadour.

This is what contemplation leads to. Contemplation of what? Of perfect femininity? Of beauty? The Lady, perversely, if we like, displays herself, following this scopic drive of which we said that it governs her (cf. chapter 3): she displays nothing – but, in displaying herself, she calls out.

She is beauty, she wishes herself beautiful because she is afraid. Beauty is a stratagem; it is a veil which designates her somewhere else than where she is. It is a lure. Of course, there is no objective reason which makes it possible to say that woman is more beautiful than man. Beauty, in her, is very simply functional (in our time, in our society). And this function is that of the lure.

The effect of the beautiful on desire. . . It is namely this something which seems singularly to divide it in two at the spot where it goes on its way. For it cannot be said that desire is completely extinguished by the apprehension of beauty; it continues its journey; but it has, there more than anywhere, the feeling of lure manifested in some way by the area of dazzle and splendour where it lets itself be drawn. (Lacan, 1960)

Equally beauty screens and it castrates man: it can be refusal of the desire of man, murder; behind the image the subject languishes, out of reach. Nowhere else is this fatal pact better described than in Arab poetry (Tahar Labib Djedidi, 1974).

Udrite love is founded indeed on a pact: woman, the **only one**, shall be loved until death and in chastity; 'woman's beauty incites us to chastity.' Double subversion consequently, if man who desires all women by vocation renounces them for the only one.

It is also true of the brotherly pact. For this 'ethical relation is not founded on the absence of desire, despite what both wish to be believed. Much rather on the refusal to give in to it, otherwise the relation would not only be destined to death but stillborn. If desire was not smouldering somewhere, the symbolic play, no longer nourished, would fall through. But because desire is there, potent, the brother and the sister genially achieve the impossible: Nietzsche and his sister; Claudel and his sister (so truly beautiful, as only some mad women are, that one should wonder about that kind of beauty); Goethe and Cornelia. . .

Cornelia, as Goethe himself admitted, was not properly speaking beautiful; but she had such 'a moral beauty that her eyes shone with it in an extraordinary way'; and her whole person expressed such a 'depth' that her brother could only 'adore her'. It was obviously the reflection of a soul which was in question in this body! It was hardly a body, even though it was 'tall and well built'. Can a reflection live long? Men did not fancy Cornelia. Perhaps also she thought herself not beautiful enough to be a woman. Yet Goethe wished her beautiful in spite of the refutations which transpire even in his words. Beauty is a reflection, a veil, a screen which hides the nakedness of woman. 'Do not uncover the nakedness of woman; it is the nakedness of your father.'

If woman and man have come to a settlement (a settlement which does not settle anything, but it does not matter here) so that woman is the phallus and man has it, then the sister owes it to herself to be beautiful for her brother. She owes it to him, as he owes it to her to be a genius. Thus she veils the nothing which is unbearable for the beloved; out of modesty she clothes herself in it. The narcissistic woman goes further since it is to and from herself that she thus indicates and hides her own vacuity: she is therefore very unhappy; this beauty in which she wants others to believe, she does not believe in; but certainly, she is attached to it all the same. In connection with the Giraffe, to whom this thought brings me back, I must add that she dares not wear a skirt. She would like to, to prove herself completely feminine. 'But, with a skirt on, I feel naked,' she says.

It is in the words of all men and women analysands (with the exceptions that I am going to mention) that it is seen that beauty is a **function**. According to these words their mother is beautiful. It is not always the case that these same words present us with a father who is a genius. We must conclude from it that the beauty of the mother is the phallus of the father (and therefore he has it) and, at the same time, the veil which hides the nakedness of the father from the son and the daughter. When by chance the mother is ugly (as is the case for a woman analysand) and the father beautiful, **rien ne va plus**. She does not know if she must choose to be **ugly** like her mother or **passive** like her father. Fortunately, the father was a painter, and the analysand became one.

We know what deal the beautiful Alcibiades proposed to his ugly but genius of a lover: genius for beauty. But for the one who is not taken in, beauty is also the last veil, the limit, beyond which there is nothing left, other than the desire of nothing – the desire of desire.

Beautiful and **of genius** are adjectives which have here no psychological reality. Just as the **mad** mother, the **sick** father, the **small** husband and the **bearded** other (the members of the paradigmatic family of the narcissistic daughter) are accompanied by adjectives of the order of the Homeric **fiery** and **haughty**.

Genius, beauty: settlement between brother and sister, we have said; yes, to avoid the Oedipus and castration. Of course, the fraternal Oedipus is still an Oedipus. Procustes, when her brother dies, mourns her father. But why did this mourning have to wait for the death of the brother, and of that brother? No other member of the family therefore could touch her so radically through their death. Her mother's death a few years earlier had left her unmoved.

Any fraternal relation permits an avoidance of the Oedipus and of castration, whether this relation is hetero- or homosexual. It is such a relation which founds the hippie communities or the religious or political communities. In this sense Hegel, like Goethe, like Musil, all are a-social; they deny the necessity for man and woman of accepting castration and their desire of man and woman in order to reach the real in separation. All three dream of the couple as one; now, that couple calls for death. The wisest, Goethe, seems to know it; but the dream is tenacious and rigid like some glass where his whole work appears to be caught up.

A similar taking up of fraternal incest in a work of literature is the basis of the Manns' novels from uncle to nephew (see above, pp. 85–86). More specifically in *The Holy Sinner* the incest committed by the brother and the sister only happens after the father's death. Equally the murder of a dog by the lover comes to signify that through the animal it is the father who is killed a second time.

Neither the slaughter nor the incest are the equivalent of an Oedipal resolution, however. In contrast the analytic relation, as it is also spoken love, strongly maintains separation. The analyst signifies through his interventions or silences that his desire does not coincide with that of the analysand. In that sense, this relation is quite exactly the reverse of the brotherly relation. Not only is there no encounter which has for ever already happened, in a mythical parental past immediately recognized by the brothers as founding; but the analysand learns that there never will be an encounter. As there never is meeting of two desires in a single one, because there is no 'sexual relation'.

Woman is extremely interested in the myth of the fraternal relation for it allows her to avoid castration from the start and saves her from division – apparently! She finds a half again, her half. Thus she is deeply attached to this cult. The trap, when the brother is truly somewhat of a genius, is practically unavoidable; the sister has enough to keep her occupied, that is to say to fill herself, she who was 'vacant'. One day, she discovers that she's 'been had'. Who possesses her? She is not full in any case, quite the contrary; and as far as unity is concerned, if someone reaches it, it is perhaps the brother. Is it the brother who possesses her? But she, then, would be reduced to zero. Thus Cornelia who 'had not reached her unity, nor was capable of reaching it' (so her brother says) dies **prematurely**, whilst Agatha commits suicide.

The brother constituting the ideal – an impossible ideal, since in any case a woman is not a man by virtue of the postulate which founds this relation – the sister identifies with him before knowing that she could in the event have a desire stronger than this ideal. If he writes, she writes; if he paints, she paints; or better still, there is only one hand to write and to paint, the one writing or painting through the hand of the other. Thus all difference is abolished. The sister considers that her brother's work is hers as well, and rightly so. Does she not know better than he does what he wanted to say or do? Here he is then, this child of the father, for ever refused; she has got him: it is the brother's work. One knows the abusive behaviour of Nietzsche's sister in relation to his work. But she considered herself to be the rightful depositary of it and – who knows? – the author. A single hand to paint; a single hand to write, and – maybe – a single penis to make love.

There is no need, in order to explain this mutual identification (which would be better called mimeticization) and the murderous effects of jealousy, to speak of **Reaktionsbildung**, of 'reaction formation' (following Freud): a relation which is characterized by jealousy where 'the rival becomes a love object through narcissistic choice of the same'.

The case of Lavallée, presented by Paul Lemoine (1974), shows the process at work in this fraternal identification:

His sister, the ninth of fifteen children, was born when La-vallée was a year and a half. It is she who appears as the key to the drama of his female identification. He himself is convinced of it. 'If I accepted Lilette, I would at the same time accept mummy and daddy.' It is a question for him of keeping intact the place of wanted child (falsely, since it is through identification with his sister that he meets the maternal desire). . . One night he had this dream: he went hunting and killed a deer; he put the corpse in the cellar. He hid it therefore and feels very guilty; guilty of having killed daddy and of having profoundly cheated him. . .

Keeping the dead, putting it aside, only serves to secure the equilibrium of a subject for whom what matters above all is keeping a place intact. He will be able to repeat the same scenario indefinitely in such clandestine shapes that he will be completely taken in. The analysis recently revealed this scenario, it is the impregnating of his mother and the identification with this mother: identification with the pregnancy; identification with the child.

From ten o'clock in the morning I must, he says, fill my stomach, be pregnant. I must have had the desire to be pregnant when Lilette came.

He then tells a nightmare from his youth: he finds himself in a well of shit and cannot get out of it. Lavallée still now lies on a raincoat spread on his bed and he experiences with delight the warmth of his excrements. (cf. chapter 5, p. 121, concerning the 'mud' in Michel Tournier)

He who goes hunting loses his place and, meanwhile, the father does his job in the mother's bed. The corpse of the deer is the father killed by Lavallée in spirit as well as the foetus with which he himself would like to be pregnant in order to be close to his mother and in his mother in place of his father, following a regressive process of identification with the sister (whom he, Lavallée, has swallowed up [avalée]).

This is where the mechanism of the fraternal relation can be seen laid bare: for the brother it is a question of surreptitiously driving the father away from his place near the mother and also near the sister. If the fraternal incest 'settles' things for the sister, it does not settle them any less for the brother.

The effects of such a fraternal relation are disastrous: sexual quasi-impotence, prolonged virginity, then premature ejaculation; incapacity to work, for the brother, and both remaining single. Disastrous as well in the case (it is an extreme case, says Musil apologetically) when the couple does not pretend and faces the incest. (Although it is not clear, on reading it, whether the incest is consummated or not.) Disastrous for Antigone whom it leads to suicide. It is only in Hegel's philosophy and in Goethe's work that it is conceived as perfect and even – for Goethe – happy.

The couple of Macarie and the Astronomer in *Wilhelm Meister's Years of Travel* is perfection of perfection. They are not brother and sister – at least I do not remember that they are – but they would deserve to be. So the blessed Macarie possesses astronomy or astrology from birth. The

Astronomer himself recognizes it and comes to the conclusion that 'not only did she carry the whole solar system in her, but she moved in spirit as an integral part of this system', a harmony for which Goethe creates a new word: 'Symphronic'. It is more or less what Theresa says of women's knowledge and men's science. So Macarie knows, by virtue of what she is: an integral part of the universe. This is expressed by the fact that she is subjected to the same laws which make the planets move and rule the shifts in the sky.

Ever since Persephone, enslaved by Hades, was forced to make periodical sojourns in Hell, one no longer knows if she thus brought about the seasons in nature or if she obeyed the natural laws of periodicity. Her mother Demeter, at least, was not subjected to these laws. There never is a way, with myths, of unearthing the causes which they spirit away.

In any case, woman happens to be biologically subjected to cycles and when a man makes an hysterical female identification, it is periodicity which serves as unitary trait. I shall mention one case only here – because the theme will be taken up in the next chapter – which Dr Naquet communicated to me during a conversation. It was about a priest who came to see him at the beginning of his career ('quite long already,' he says and he adds: 'it must be that this case struck me') about a 'moon sickness'. He claimed to have an attack every twenty-eight days. It seems that it was a matter of hysterical epilepsy of a female nature which could lead us to posit that periodicity in itself is symptomatic in man.

Through her belonging, woman somehow knows. Her desire is to be. She participates in creation. But that is also how she is once more divided. It is the dividing of women, their suffering and their **jouissance**.

For man the dividing line goes between woman and him, we have said; and it is her, as creature, whom he questions. Woman does not question man. And yet Macarie needs the Astronomer in order to know that she knows. In return, man's science would be science of nothing if it did not encounter this knowing.

One sees here how easily the sister, who was beauty, can – arguing from her knowledge – have pretentions to science, and how easily the play of identification is triggered, through which she grants herself the phallus. The brother is thus dispossessed without the sister being, for all that, provided for, except in the ideal society of Goethe. It is a struggle which was covered by a beautiful dream. But everything can be used by woman to avoid castration. How could she have let this brother escape? How would they not believe that nature had placed them next to each other on purpose, in a relation of perfect convenience, by virtue of a pre-established parental harmony – parental and even cosmic – in order for them to unite and for creation to be thus perfect? A relation of a nostalgic and therefore regressive kind; its participants do not reach maturity.

The perversion of the fraternal relation has its maximum effect in twins who may be taken as the partners of an accomplished fraternal relation. 'There were two years between Klaus and his sister Erika,' Michel Tournier tells us, 'and yet a triumphant tour of the USA in 1927 led them to be known as the Mann twins.' Similarly Goethe and his sister, by Goethe's own admission, experienced themselves as twins; and also Lucille and Chateaubriand, the latter of whom writes: 'The story is told of two twins who were ill together, healthy together, and who, when they were apart, could closely see what was happening to the other one: it is my story and that of Lucille, with the difference that the twins died on the same day and I have survived my sister.' With the difference, also, that he was four years younger than she and that they were not twins.

Brothers and sisters wish themselves twins, indeed. The twin state expresses the ideal of their relation (cf. the case of Philiberte above, p. 37); the two births are reduced to a single one. All historical difference is denied for the benefit of the simple grammatical opposition brother/sister. It is opposition in place of difference. Whether they are of the same or of a different sex, they define themselves from the start as he/she: masculine/feminine; big/small, etc., without their own respective identities being in the least engaged in that organization. In other words, the heshe runs in neutral. It is the anti-analytic relation par excellence, the perfect symmetrical relation, lure itself.

However, the fraternal relation, particularly the twin relation, from the start, places the couple beyond that limit where the natural bonds of love provide alibis for the one who wants to live 'in the service of the good' according to the formula already quoted, by which Lacan characterizes all morality, even the highest, which is invested in satisfaction and not in desire. In that, this relation is unique and, from that fact, irreplaceable. Who loses a brother has only one thing left: to die after having buried him. That is what Antigone does. Agatha is more 'savage', dying after consummation of love. Antigone saves a unique, irreplaceable brother from dispersion, from nowhere, from asymbolic death. 'After the death of a spouse, another can replace him,' says Sophocles' Antigone. 'After the death of a son, another can give me a second one; but I can no longer hope for the birth of a brother.' And yet she has other brothers. It must be that, compared with this one, they do not count. And could she really not have another one (cf. Lacan, 1960)?

Procustes says nothing else. She had, it is true, two husbands and several lovers. But she only had this brother. Had they been two or more, each would have been irreplaceable as having happened before any choice and any personal action, before the beginning (outside of duration) of her history. Each one – the brother and the sister – free of each other, and yet tied since before history, because born of one and the same matrix and of a couple presumed united for this aim.

The fraternal Oedipus is more difficult to resolve than the other one, but equally – provided it is pushed to its limit – it makes the subject touch on this between-two-deaths which goes from the death of desire to the other death and which is the harsh law of analysis. Anti-analytic, therefore, as lure, because it is then at the service of the good; but close to analytic resolution as ultimate lure, after which the desire of desire can begin to last (cf. Lacan, 1960).

5

The hermaphrodite

If someone had told me that the absence
of another would make me doubt existence,
how I would have sniggered! . . . To exist,
what does it mean? It means to be outside,
sister ex. . .

Michel Tournier, *Friday or the Other Island*
('Ex-sistence' is the spelling that Lacan's
teaching has led us to adopt)

THE manifestation, or the root, or the model of this
aspiration to unity – which is accompanied by mysticism
in the brother/sister couple* – are easily traceable in myths (do
we ever know with myths?), but also in the religions where
twins are gods; and elsewhere in hermaphroditism. **The failure
of the sexual relation as far as a possible realization of unity is
concerned** leads the individual to satisfy himself on his own
and to achieve the '**coincidentia oppositorium**'. It is the
same coincidence that the hysteric attempts to achieve when
she bends in an arc. 'The great hysterical attack evokes at
the same time a bisexual coital manifestation', Freud notes
(1908).

PRESIDENT SCHREBER

President Schreber (all the quotations from President Schreber are taken from his autobiographical *Memoirs of my*

---

* In that sense it can be said with Jung that the unconscious is mystical. Still,
one mustn't go as far as believing what the mystics say. One must believe
them. But not believe in what they say: for it is the fruit of an experience,
and as far as experience is concerned, to each his own. I take up here,
distorting it somewhat, the Lacanian distinction between **believing it** and
believing in it.

Nervous Illness (1903)* – in quite another register, for he is not an hysteric, it seems – says exactly the same thing: 'I have to imagine myself as man and woman in one person having intercourse with myself.' God demands it. He demands a constant state of **jouissance**. Before being a demand, however, it was for Schreber only an 'idea', 'imposed' as if from outside in the shape of a dream, or half a dream; an idea worded thus: 'It really must be rather pleasant to be a woman succumbing to intercourse.' It is the very dream of the Giraffe (cf. chapter 2) and perfectly symmetrical. But it is only a dream. Mircéa Eliade (1962) reminds us that it has a counterpart. The hermaphrodite 'represented in Antiquity an ideal situation and an attempt was made to actualize it spiritually through the intervention of rituals; but if a child showed signs of hermaphroditism at birth, he was put to death by his own parents'.

This 'idea' which imposes itself thus on President Schreber one morning, the realization of which he does not wish in any way – for what he wants is to be a full man, a president: exactly what his recent nomination at the Dresden Court of Appeal tells him that he is, summons him to be – has been taking shape for a few weeks to the point where it has brought about transformations in his body in which he believes. I shall say about him what I said earlier about Theresa: if he believes in it, I believe him. One cannot doubt the word of President Schreber when he solemnly and repeatedly summons, implores, doctors and experts to come and observe the signs of femininity which affect his body: soft woman skin, breasts which swell and unswell, female bosom, and network of voluptuous nerves which runs under the skin of the whole body, so that he experiences this voluptuousness all over and not only in the sexual organ and its immediate vicinity.

[* The published French and English translations of Schreber differ slightly. All quotations in this chapter are from the English edition (1955), except on pp.109–10, where we have translated directly from the French edition (1975), to preserve the significance Lemoine-Luccioni attaches to certain words.]

I would at all times be prepared to submit my body to medical examination for ascertaining whether my assertion is correct, that my whole body is filled with nerves of voluptuousness from the top of my head to the soles of my feet, such as is the case only in the adult female body, whereas in the case of a man, as far as I know, nerves of voluptuousness are only found in and immediately around the sexual organs.

I will even go as far as to say that these words deserve more due consideration, since they focus on a difference between male pleasure and female pleasure, which is not negligible and which is above all described here for the first time.

Lethe (cf. chapter 3), who was falling from her high horse since the start of her first periods and pathologically **fell** asleep at any time of the day, describes her pleasure in quite similar terms. 'I have started again with François. It's wonderful. It's not that I have so many orgasms. But I have pleasure for two or three days afterwards. It's euphoric. It remains **in my whole body**. For my husband it's pure profit. Well, I feel good all the time. Of course I have to make love again after a few days. . .' Lethe is fifty; she has had thirty years of married life and total frigidity. She has discovered pleasure with young men the same age as her daughters, whom she meets at Vincennes University where she started studying at the same time as she started in psychotherapy after being asleep the whole length of her life as a woman.

It is also when he is over fifty that Schreber, although happily married, it seems, is faced with this crisis which has all the characteristics of a mystical experience: **illumination** (properly and figuratively speaking), ontological mutation and upheaval in the natural order of the universe. I borrow these points from Mircéa Eliade (1962) who writes:

A few corollaries result from this pan-Indian metaphysic of Light and in particular: 1) the most adequate revelation of divinity happens through Light; 2) those who have reached a high level of spirituality – that is to say, in Indian terms, have achieved or at least approached the situation of a 'freed one' or of a Buddha – are equally able to irradiate

The divine rays of President Schreber and his suns tell the same story, and when they 'penetrate' his body, they give him a 'voluptuousness sufficient for souls . . . without real sexual excitement' and make him feel 'a general bodily well-being'. When he is kept a male, in other words when he is refused **éviration** ['emasculation'], he is condemned to physical deterioration and dementia: his 'existence' (that is the word he uses) is threatened. What is therefore in question for him, as for all mystics, is whether to live as the wife of God or as a castrated man.

The parallel path of identification without copulation does not always lead to mystical or pseudo-mystical delusion. On the contrary, in so-called normal man and woman, copulation does not go without a kind of identification and sex change. In coitus, as in **couvade**, what man seeks to find is perhaps participation – natural to woman – in the great cycles, the great periods of creation. Fliess, as we know, believed he had discovered a male periodicity: 23 days instead of 28, and the psychoanalyst Jean Guir says: 'These phenomena of periodicity incited Freud to transform their content into the diabolical notion of repetition which will end up later in the death instinct' (Guir, 1975-6).

To confine ourselves to pregnancy, all the testimonies of a Groddeck confirm that of Schreber: man has a wish for pregnancy which is expressed by a swelling of such or such part of the belly, vomiting and other palpable somatic manifestations. I have mentioned myself, in chapter 2, cases of identification with pregnancy, from which it may be concluded that the identification at work in the wish for a sex change, wish to 'show himself' or to 'pass for' as Schreber says, really affects man's body.

Moreover, do we not know that it can be seen with a naked eye, in some cases, whether a man has made a female identification? 'You carry your mother here', a slightly shaman therapist says one day to Claude, while touching his belt. Claude is left-handed; he is all round and his skin is so fine (like Schreber's) that he gets scratched all the time. He then screams like a woman, which you do not expect from this being, otherwise perfectly in his place of man in society. The voice, with its double register, often betrays this female incorporation in men, as we know. And yet Claude does not seem to be an hysteric any more than Schreber. Identification serves them only as a false peg, as a return effect of a missed encounter with the Other. The child is then called upon by man as well as woman to occupy the ever vacant place. . .

It follows from the above that, for one sex as well as the other, the child may be what comes in the place of the Other. Which does not signify that he is enough in that place. For, from the moment of the sexual act, as far as castration is concerned, the game is up. What clearly appears, in the symptomatology of the neuroses and the psychoses, is penis envy in women, despite their claims of hatred; and the wish to procreate in men, despite their contempt for femininity. Those motifs provided by the great myths can be found in the 'personal' myths of neurotics. Like the Hungarian bus driver mentioned by Lacan (1956-7) who had been living as 'quite a normal man until an accident and above all until the X-rays which (supposedly) brought about a traumatic hysteria from which the latent fantasy of pregnancy was discovered'. The child in that case was well hidden, but the X-ray brought it into the open.

Groddeck considers that every man has a fantasy of pregnancy, a 'child hidden somewhere'. In every case, it is a question for man of spiriting the Other away, in the event woman, in order to make her reappear in the shape of a child. This is how President Schreber describes the phenomenon.

Something like the conception of Jesus Christ by an Immaculate Virgin – i.e. one who never had intercourse with a man – happened in my own body. Twice at different times . . . I had a female genital organ, although a poorly developed one, and in my body felt quickening like the first signs of life of a human embryo: by a divine miracle God's nerves corresponding to male seed had been thrown into my body; in other words fertilization had occurred.

Schreber pays dearly for this frenzied wish for mutation and so does Claude, who says clearly that he no longer recognizes

himself and that he never recognizes anybody: 'I don't identify faces', he repeats. And, as could be expected, he is a
painter. I imagine that the world is, as it were, thrown into
his face in its newness at every moment, precisely because he
does not recognize it.

As for President Schreber, he lived amongst a population
of ghosts. In the people around him, he thought he recognized
all kinds of people more or less invented, who mixed up all
countries and all times. To identify no one and to identify
everyone with everyone; to recognize no one and to think you
recognize everyone is the same phenomenon. Besides, Claude
always thinks he has just walked by X or Y in the street, and
one can be sure that he is mistaken.

In this failure of recognizing which turns the others into
'botched-up beings' without true consistency, the subject
himself is caught. He does not see himself. Claude bumps into
everything and Schreber speaks of his ability to 'picture' himself other than he is; and, for instance, he 'pictures' a woman's
behind on himself, so that God will not be too disappointed
at night. He maintains, with the greatest precision and the
firmest decision, that these pictures are quite convincing
for him, as real as possible. His analysis of the picture and
of the design is remarkable. In connection with recognizing,
it is necessary, I believe, to quote everything that Schreber
says and which leads to the development of the picture/
design.

*I chose the very simple case of a man I know and whom I
would happen to meet. Upon seeing him, this thought arises
in me quite naturally and automatically: this man is called
Schneider, or else: here is Schneider. Now, as soon as this
thought is formulated, there starts resounding in my nerves a
'why then' or a 'why because'. If someone were to start asking
this kind of question to another person, within the context of
ordinary relations between people, it is likely that they would
get the following answer: Why? This is a stupid question,
this man is called Schneider, that's all there is to it. And yet
my nerves cannot and could not be content with adopting the
simple solution which consisted in avoiding these questions
in that way. The issue of the* **cause,** *quite strangely posited*

*in this case, snatches my nerves into a kind of mechanical
gearing and they exhaust themselves in unceasing repetitions
. . . If perhaps, at first, my nerves are brought to give this
answer: well, this man is called Schneider because* **his father**
*is also called Schneider, they cannot find any peace in such a
trivial answer. And a whole series of enquiries and research
about the foundations and the* **origin of people's names** *gets
under way. (my emphasis)*

The sex change is thus directly linked to the impossibility of
taking on the name after the father; and Schreber chooses
then to return to the origin of names, that is to say to the one
who, through an act of spontaneous generation, is supposed
to have begotten the first man, without going through the other, woman, copulation. From which point Schreber manages
to systematize his delusion; he finds the simple solution which
consists in letting himself be penetrated by God in order to
engender a new race. In order to do this, he must become a
woman. The problem is that the conjuring trick comes back
like a boomerang. He had the woman; she was his wife and a
reciprocal love united them. All that remained for him then
was to become God and it was no more difficult than to become
a woman. But it is precisely (becoming God himself) what he
was not entitled to, what he **could** not allow himself to claim.
As for her, his wife **could** not give him a live child – it is a fact,
and it appears to be contingent. Neither **could** he therefore
become a father in that way, kill his father somehow, in that
way. Finally, his father incarnated the law in its absolute; and
thus **could** not die.

Lacan's teaching throws some light on all these impossi-
bilities against which Schreber came up. Schreber cannot
add the extra **I** which the real confrontation with his father
would have allowed him to trace, constituting at the same
time the series of numbers and names of his genealogy. Failing
this extra **I**, genealogies and centuries collapsing are merged
into synchrony and Schreber finds himself sucked towards
the zero which precedes all origin, all numerical series. As
he cannot reasonably accept being a zero and as he cannot
consecrate himself **primo motore** [prime mover] and **primo
fattore** [prime doer] for the reasons I have given, the only

place left for him to occupy is that of woman, next to this First One, postulated outside of creation.

The conjuring trick consists precisely in by-passing the Oedipus. It is a question here again of escaping castration, of **not making an attempt against the father**, who, like God, incarnates the law for Schreber and as such remains unkillable – and of begetting without begetting while begetting, since as we said his couple is childless. From which it can be said echoing Freud that 'the unconscious is destiny'. I shall restrict myself here with taking up the account that Myriam Pécaut gave of Reik's book (Reik, 1946):

*The rites of **couvade** are accompanied by tests during which wounds are inflicted on the father by the members of the tribe, attenuated forms, according to Reik, of emasculation, substitutes for castration. The last transformation, it seems, of the relation between the father and the new-born, this trial by blood reveals the full extent of the drama which is played for man at the birth of a child, a drama which brings into play the very question of his existence . . . For what is in question is indeed knowing who will die or who will die first, father or son. Renouncing the power that the father holds of destroying the child, in the absolute, can only be the result of a profound mutation which does not go without the detour of a symbolization: that of the institution of a succession of generations. Abraham, in suspending the murder of his son, accepts that the child shall not die before the father. . .*

In by-passing the obstacle of castration, Schreber fails to **knot** the 'loops' of the Imaginary and the Symbolic (Lacan, 1974-5) by a crossing of the Real which would keep them together. Hence his imaginary universe floats, held through his sole belief. The imaginary, which offers to our contemplation (ours and Kant's) the starry sky above our heads and the internal law inside, in a consensus ratified by common sense, creates two suns instead of one in the eyes of Schreber; a valley filled with a luxurious vegetation or a desert, according to his mood, and inside, unbearable bites or voluptuousness, according to the fate of a merciless struggle. He is alone, absolutely alone in knowing all of that.

The crossing of the real is this death which we risk simply in agreeing to recognize that the Other (and specifically the father for the son) prevents us from living by being there. It is not enough to substitute oneself for the Father, or to take his place, or to take the place of a grandfather, as was apparently done in some tribes where the son received a name only at the death of the grandfather, as if he had to wait for a place to be vacant in order to be recognized as living. It is necessary to replace this principle of substitution by that of generation (Lévi-Strauss, 1962), and to recognize that there is not always an equal number of human beings, once and for all, but that it is necessary to submit to time and to admit this extra one which appears, which comes to make a knot, the knot of castration and of existence. There is death indeed, but it is for everyone, for the father as well as the son, with the exception perhaps of the Father of the primal Tribe, this mythical being of which it is said that 'it is always necessary that there is at least 1' who does not accept the phallic law, for there to be 'some all' who know about it.

One must not be surprised that neither a woman nor anyone can stand in for this Other who delivers the one into a certain existence, if what has been called the Oedipus is not resolved. The Other in all its manifestations will always be missed and sexual life compromised. Therefore Schreber returns to the most undifferentiated drive: being penetrated, absorbing, vomiting, shitting, all through the intermediary of rays which can fill him up with God as well as with Flechsig, his doctor. That is what he calls being a woman. That is at least what a man becomes when he wants to change into a woman: a psychotic.

Schreber could not take the place of his father, because he was for him the non-castrated Father; he could not properly speaking be President in spite of his nomination; he therefore could in no way be God. There was only one place left for him, that of the wife of God, even if he had to sacrifice his beloved wife; which he did.

However, the miracle he talks about so much is properly speaking this amazing **voluptuousness** that the delusion obtains for him, 'however botched up' it may be in my opinion. (I take up here, in a different context, a word which is dear to

him.) If he did not experience such voluptuousness – wholly
feminine indeed – suffering would get the better of him. But
above all, he would not be able to believe in his mission, his
truth. You cannot refuse a heavenly state.

TERRE-FLEUR [EARTH-FLOWER]

It was a young male analysand of nineteen who threw some
light for me on Schreber's heavenly state. Terre-Fleur was
sent to me by an acupuncturist with whom he was doing yoga,
after an eight-day psychotic episode and a stay in hospital.
That is all I knew about him when I saw this tall thin man
with white skin, doe's eyes and a long Jewish nose: the head
and body of Christ; a woman's smile; much deference in his
demeanour; a beautiful voice. A virgin, as I soon learnt, and
falling in love easily with girls to whom he immediately speaks
of life involvement and who must necessarily present high
intellectual qualities.

Terre-Fleur despises his father and his three brothers.
He bitterly reproaches his father for not being a writer,
a philosopher or a musician (a violinist, for example). In
brief, 'he's a wanker'. He is in business and travels abroad
a lot. He has intelligent friends whom Terre-Fleur admires.
The brothers are noisy and 'complete wankers'. He does not
reproach his mother for anything. She does everything well.
She is intelligent and she has taste. It can be seen that he splits
mankind in two: men on the one hand, contemptible; and
women on the other, worthy of every devotion. But he has a
male ideal (the philosophy teacher, friend of his father) who
is the very person he would like to become, whereas he is only
poorly gifted in that respect and his 'illness' makes working
difficult ('his brothers prevent him from working, of course,
these idiots!') and it happens that most of the girls he meets
and who would like to sleep with him are not interesting
'intellectually'.

It is exactly a girl of this kind whom he meets after a
few months of therapy (I do not say that it is necessarily the
result of therapy). So he sleeps with Zizi who is ugly and very
forward. The event does not seem to touch him very much;
no doubt because Zizi is not his sweetheart who – so beautiful
– remains out of reach. But above all because what has

taken place with a woman falls far short of his psychotic happiness.

He talked to me quite soon of his delusion, after three sessions, guessing that I knew something about it in any case. This delusion occurred in the countryside where his parents have a house and garden; Terre-Fleur feels perfectly well there. He never has any criticism, any·reproach for this place, this land, this house fixed up by his mother. He lovingly works in the garden, looks after the trees, goes for walks, visits the neighbours, etc. In one word, it is the only place where it seems that he can live; even though, his mother being a foreigner, it is to the country of his mother that he dreams of going.

His delusion then occurred in the countryside, but after a stay abroad where he had already 'felt strange'. He came there for the end of his holidays, alone, as he often did for a weekend or at other times. I repeat that he is always very happy there, excited by what he does and in good shape physically. This time, he was found wandering – by some neighbours – much thinner, not knowing the day or the time or the place. Lost in short. But happy.

He frequently went back over this delusion. He is the one who used the word, as well as the word mysticism in this connection. When he told me that he wanted to go back to this country house, but that he was afraid, even after a year of therapy and success (he passed his exams when he had failed the year before; he slept with a girl; he has plans for intellectual, professional and skilled training at Vincennes University), I asked him why he was afraid, since the delusion was so pleasant. 'Yes, I know,' he said, 'a lot of people told me that it was wonderful to experience such a state and many would like to get to it (for reasons of space I have not mentioned his paranoid tendencies, even though they are of some importance): but I was almost starving. I don't sleep, I don't eat, I don't know when it's time to do this or that. I don't even know who I am. Then I'm afraid.' Indeed he loses weight when he goes through those states to the point of being a shadow of his former self. He prefers then to be 'followed' by someone (myself, in the event); to do his work-out every morning to strengthen his body (in case the mind weakens), to

eat as healthily and rationally as possible in order not to lose
weight, or have diarrhoea; in brief, he drives himself hard to
be fit to work, to read, to think, to prepare his exams, because
he is proud and he wants to succeed. **So, no delusion.** As far
as he is able, he will not allow it to himself. Nevertheless, he
hesitates: don't you think I'm strong enough now to. . . ?

To what? What is he asking me? For it is immersion and
fusion which are in question. What his bliss is lacking is being
guaranteed by God and supported by a new ordering of the
universe so that Terre-Fleur will not die of his delusion. In the
event, it is more a goddess of vegetation who might guarantee
him. What he is lacking therefore is the ability to systematize
this delusion.

FRIDAY

It is a literary work once more which is going to throw some
light on a clinical case: from Terre-Fleur's delusion, we go on
to Tournier's *Friday*. But before coming to *Friday*, I would
like to mention something that Michel Tournier himself said,
on the radio, in August 1975, in answer to someone who was
surprised by the complete absence of women in this novel: 'It
is on the contrary a great feminine cosmic novel . . . woman
is the island; she is the sister, the wife, the mother, everything. . .' And in connection with his work, he added: 'I think
that our times are mystical.' If we add the word **mystical** to
the words **great feminine cosmic novel**, we obtain a complete
formulation of the Schreberian epic.

It is quite true that the island is the woman for Robinson.
The proof is that he is jealous of his black companion, Friday
(him, the redhead), when he discovers that the white man-
drake flowers, which were growing in the earth fecundated by
his sperm, grow one morning with brown stripes, 'streaked'.
Proof that the earth has been polluted by the sperm of the
other. So, the earth is a beloved woman and, lying on her,
Robinson experiences a perfect voluptuousness. But the child
he will have – for he too is stirred by a wish to procreate – will
fall from the sky or the sun, one morning. He will not come out
of the earth. It will be a red-haired boy like himself or golden
like a 'ray detached from the sun'. An unexpected ship will
leave him on the quietened sea . . . a child from the Sun-God;

not a child from the Earth: Thursday, son of Jupiter. The novelesque thread can then be called a miracle. If the child is not engendered by the mother, he can only be the product of a miracle, indeed.

Woman is not absent from this novelesque myth. But precisely only as a mythical being. However different this scenario might be from that of Schreber or Terre-Fleur, what is in question for a man is to recapture a total voluptuousness in a communion or fusion or abandon which has no other aim than this communion or fusion or abandon. Which is the interested other? There is no interested other, other than the earth, nature, creation or God. It is to be noted that God alone is a male partner here. Delusion is happy; fatal nonetheless.

Gilles Deleuze, in his afterword to *Friday* (cf. also Deleuze, 1969) describes the phenomenon in the same terms as Schreber: 'Consciousness has become not only an internal phosphorescence of things, but also a flame in their heads, a light above each one, a "flying I". In this light something else appears, airy double of each thing. . . That is what the novel excels in describing: in each case the extraordinary birth of the erected double.' It could not be put better; and the explanation given by Deleuze is valid for Schreber as well as for Robinson. If there is delusion, it is because others presided over the organization of the world of objects and over the transitive relations between these objects, and they no longer do.

The absence of others – the foreclosure of the signifier which would have made them subsist – results in the universe collapsing into a world where the subject suffers a thousand unbearable tortures against which, as we have seen, he constructs his heavenly delusion, when he manages it. And if he does not manage to, he constructs himself as he can, with somewhere in him this camouflaged, sealed, built-up, mastered hole, in the manner of Terre-Fleur. (In the manner also of Percival, cf. Bateson, 1961, and of a whole category of sports people who do not want to let the pain go through their body and believe that they can muzzle it.)

Robinson goes through the disturbing dusk and the rut of an end of the world where 'everything is implacable' and everything is 'wounding', according to the schema of psycho-

sis brought out by Lacan. It is because he refuses to go through
the detour of others to structure the world. He widens the
hole instead of building it, and he draws out his **jouissance**.
He becomes a 'Robinson of the Sun in the Island which
has become Solar'. He is a Schreber who wins the game and
carries creation in his wake. 'His final aim is the encounter
of libido with free elements, the discovery of a cosmic energy
or of a great elementary Health. . .' Robinson is young for
eternity.

What then is the point of a child? Is elementary happiness
not sufficient? 'Others are indispensable, but they can be
replaced,' writes Tournier. Thursday happens to be there
miraculously, to replace Friday who betrayed Robinson and
embarked on the Whitebird. What if the miracle had not
taken place?

The novel is a continuous miracle: just at the time when the
Whitebird, intruding in Robinson's world, brought illness
and time back to him and threatened to carry the insular
innocent into the 'degrading and fatal whirlwind of time', a
child gives immortality back to him.

THE PREGNANT MAN

Lacan underlines the fact that the desire for procreation lies
'at the bottom of Schreber's symptomatology'. Certainly, as
he wishes to be mother in order to be father, like Robinson.
But it is a conjuring trick which only succeeds in novels and
myths.

Claude Lévi-Strauss discovers the universality of male
procreation in *L'homme nu* [*The Naked Man*, 1971], at least
as far as America is concerned. 'The theme of the pregnant
man occupies a considerable area in North America . . . it
appears to be spread even more widely in South America. . .'
It is always a question of a demiurge who has no wife and
who 'hides' his child in his knee or his elbow, in the shape of
an abscess for example. Or else **he gives himself** the child by
sticking his penis in his elbow. No doubt it would be easy to
find this same theme in other continents.

This same theme of the pregnant man is found in Groddeck;
it inevitably contains a form of procreation from which woman

is excluded; and a desire to create, or recreate the universe or a new race.

And even, if one is to believe Aeschylus, it is against woman that man thus intends to work.

> *You won the ancient goddesses over with wine*
> *And so destroyed the orders of an elder time*

says the coryphaeus to Phoebus Apollo who wants to save in Orestes the murderer of his mother and the avenger of his father. What does Apollo reply?

> *The mother is no parent of that which is called*
> *her child, but only nurse of the new-planted seed*
> *that grows. The parent is he who mounts. A stranger she*
> *preserves a stranger's seed, if no god interferes.*
> *I will show you proof of what I have explained. There*
> *can be a father without any mother. There she stands,*
> *the living witness, daughter of Olympian Zeus,*
> *she who was never fostered in the dark of the womb*
> *yet such a child as no goddess could bring to birth.*

Victory of the father against matriarchy; institution of a new order which is not that of blood. A woman, Athene, because she is the father's daughter, declares herself for men and tips the vote in favour of Orestes. It is thus the alliance of a woman who has sided with men which completes the defeat of women. It sounds just like a political meeting:

> *This is a ballot for Orestes I shall cast.*
> *There is no mother anywhere who gave me birth,*
> *and, but for my marriage, I am always for the male*
> *with all my heart, and strongly on my father's side.*
> *So, in a case where the wife has killed her husband, lord*
> *of the house, her death shall not mean most to me.*

The father's daughter who came out of his forehead fully armed, loves men, but remains a virgin.

The whole of ancient history and our own are made up of this struggle: **law of the Mother or law of the Father? And whose child is the child?** If Orestes is pardoned, it is proof that in shedding his mother's blood he only shed the blood of a stranger. As for Clytemnestra, she should not have made

her husband perish. Such is the law of the father, of Phoebus
Apollo, of the Sun, of Zeus who becomes all.

> *Zeus is ether. Zeus is earth. Zeus is sky.*
> *Zeus is all and higher than all of that.*
> (Distich quoted by Dreyfus and borrowed from Clément
> d'Alexandrie).

Dreyfus, author of the introduction to the Pléiade edition,
adds in a note that mention is also made in the Heliades of
'a gold cup . . . in which the Sun crosses the Ocean, fleeing
the depths of the holy Night with black horses'. The 'dark
continent' did not start with Freud; nor the sun divinity with
Schreber or Tournier.

Two orders, therefore two laws. The law of the Father
leaves the daughter with only the hysterical choice of identification with the phallus and virginity. The law of the Mother
is twofold. Persephone is destined to female homosexuality
and rape; but the exemplary Penthesilea offers another path
to the Mother's daughter: homosexual, she certainly is; and
men are for her and her Amazons nothing but prey from
whom they get pleasure only to reject them right away; but
when Achilles' arrow shoots through Penthesilea and her
horse, nailing her to the animal in death, he discovers at the
same time that she is a woman; what a woman is. He has the
revelation of love and can renounce Patroclus. The only thing
is, Penthesilea is dead (Quintus de Smyrne, commented on
and introduced by Sainte-Beuve).

In Julien Gracq's version after Kleist, it is on the contrary
Penthesilea who puts Achilles to death, handing him over to
her wild dogs and her elephants. She then uncovers the white
chest of the warrior who had come without armour, bites
him and draws blood. She cannot survive this action: 'I am
no longer the law of the Amazons . . . I go with the one who
is here.'

From the moment when Achilles saw Penthesilea he was no
longer able to fight: he laid down his arms, literally and figuratively speaking. And from the moment when Penthesilea
went against the laws of the Amazons by choosing Achilles
amongst others and by loving him, she went mad. What made
her madness explode is not the foreclosure of the name of the

father, but the arrival of a real man. Psychosis is an effect of foreclosure, but it only appears when there also appears **in the real** the love object cancelled out through foreclosure: here, the man whom Penthesilea cannot recognize, and she changes back into a bitch. We are brought back to women's madness. As well as dying Penthesilea pays with her madness for the refusal of castration and the revelation of the real other.

For woman as for man there is no salvation outside of symbolic castration. But if the law of the Father wins out, the fate of the sons is no happier; for the Other, which the son cannot confront in the father, is also this woman from whom he does not want a child.

It is remarkable that these others whom the father, dreary little cloth-worker with an eternal cold, was not able to bring forth for Robinson, opposite his powerful mother, and whom he irrevocably lost in the person of his young sister when she died, should return in the shape of this sister during a dangerous hallucination. It is only then, after this dangerous but wonderful vision (celestial music, beautiful ship, dances and apparitions), that he forgets about these others; that he renounces them to put doubles in their place; the one most opposed to him (Friday) and the one most similar, Thursday, the little redhead.

We know that the novel finishes in a splendid pinnacle which the author qualifies as 'a solar ecstasy'. Ah! How happy President Schreber would have been reading such a novel.

Neither the solar ecstasy nor the voluptuous coupling of the man and the Island in the 'pink coomb' are questionable, although invented by a novelist. Nor the Schreberian voluptuousness nor the happy delusion of Terre-Fleur. But that the process of dehumanization in the union of man and element could have a happy outcome is quite another thing. The outcome that we know in our society is madness. The fact remains that the other side of madness is total, imperative, continuous **jouissance**; and that it appears to be female.

Would woman, if she was all – to paraphrase Lacan – be mad? That is what my thoughts stumble upon at every turn. As for man, the price to be won for him is terrible. 'Closer to death than any living being, I am at the same time closer to the very sources of sexuality,' writes Michel Tournier on the cover of his book. He also says that he is 'suspended between heaven and hell, in limbo, in effect'.

The emasculation [**éviration**] which is imposed on Schreber, or rather which he demands, accounts better for this kind of death. It is a question of a sort of unravelling of the genital drive and a redistribution of the play of the drives throughout the body. Schreber has the feeling that his sexual organs are shrinking and go up into his body to become female organs. Absurdly, he must thus renounce the component genital drive – component, since it only concerns the genital organ, in man at least – in favour of total bliss. And yet, the genital drive whose aim is procreation could have fulfilled him. It is therefore precisely because it is component and mostly component that he cannot be satisfied with it, even if it means disorganizing the whole system of drives in order to recover the totality of his libido.

In the case of Terre-Fleur, virginity spares the boy from this work of emasculation. His bliss is spontaneous. The fact that he made love a year later with a girl who desired him has not made him more active and does not seem to have triggered the genital drive. His virginity weighed on him and worried him; he felt reassured. That is all or almost all; for, after all, he was able to make love. At least he says so, he made it, even though the absence of desire made the whole thing quite dull. He says that too. He uses another tone to speak of his delusion. What must he renounce? One does not renounce **jouissance**. It is 'demanded', Schreber would say; it is an imperative. But Terre-Fleur renounces it. He prefers to become strong and take up all kinds of physical exercises to seal this overwhelming hole, to build himself and build it.

MUD

The unravelling (what I call here **unravelling**, which is the equivalent of what is called in analytic technique disintrication [**désintrication**], is the pathological process itself, when it is not the effect of transference) of the genital drive necessarily leads to regression. Robinson and Schreber are equally specific in the description of their anal life, and I do not know which one is the most sumptuous. The episode of the mud in *Friday* is well known. Schreber is less lyrical. But actually, he finds a tone which does not lack greatness to say: 'When I do empty myself . . . this act is always combined with a very strong development of soul-voluptuousness . . . the same happens when I pass water.' But he cannot help again taking up the dogmatic and mad tone which is the very one of the 'president' when he adds: '. . . symbolic meaning of the act of defecation, namely that he who entered into a special relationship to divine rays as I have is to a certain extent entitled to shit on all the world.'

'To shit on all the world' is the leitmotiv of a well-known student song. The 'president' does not have the privilege of this frantic wish to erase every shape from the surface of the earth, to suppress the old marks and to drown the world of signs in the river of his own dejections; the wish to turn the created world into mud.

Robinson's mud has for him a much more negative meaning since it marks the state beyond which he cannot degrade himself even more, unknit himself even more, without becoming not quite an animal, for man does not have that choice – but mad. From that point, he will take a run up again to reconquer the island, the Earth, but without the woman. Robinson does not want to go mad. That is how he is not. That is how Robinson is not Schreber and is not psychotic. **He does not believe in** his hallucinations: his sister is dead; she is quite dead; she cannot come back to earth. And a man, even if he identifies with his sumptuous mother, **is not** a woman; he cannot **believe** that he **is** a woman.

Reciprocally: a woman is not a mad man.

What is really the bearing of those myths and rites 'full of what ethnologists call inversion phenomena: women with a devilish penis who take the place of the usual partner of a female relation; men losing their blood when their wives are penetrated by an other . . . disguises . . . in the ritual'? (Pécaut, 1974-5). I have already referred to the small book by Marie Delcourt, *Hermaphrodite* (1958), which rigorously demonstrates the point. But exactly what point, if not, and only, that of the constant effort of identification, and of the assumption in the ritual of a (dangerous?) process whose aim is to avert danger.

That man, during his wife's pregnancy, goes through a

dangerous episode of loss of masculinity, is what we saw in chapter 2. He cuts a sorry figure, indeed, next to this powerful mother in the making who takes the place of the spouse and even more. If she has everything, the penis in her, the phallus (the child), what more can she ask of man? And in fact, she no longer asks anything of him, which results in instantly cancelling out his phallus like blowing on a candle. He has no other means, if he also wants to become in some way the father of the child about to be born, than to identify with his wife through all sorts of physiological phenomena which are the present equivalent of the ancient **couvade** (Trehowann and Colon, in Ebtinger and Renoux, 1967). Feminization which is the consequence of the momentary emasculation (or its reverse) as well as its cause.

A page from a novel expresses best the condition which is thus imposed on man and the feeling he so often has of being 'done in' or of being 'had' (Luccioni, M., 1976). In the previous pages, the wife of the protagonist has noted that their youngest daughter had her first period; when hearing the news, the father ruminates in a long internal monologue:

Half the time, you didn't even have any [periods]; each time ten months without; what luck; just like a guy. Instead you had your belly, this slow swelling, your penis substitute; but I sometimes think that it's the opposite: the penis is a baby substitute; a poor substitute, just think: you have a nine month long erection; there's something worthwhile! And then a build up of several hours and at the end an explosion of at least a quarter of an hour. Oh! No need to tell you anything: these moans, these clenched hands, your head rolling from side to side; your lips twisting; your ears burning and after this complete discharge, sometimes a few tears and this, yes, recognition.

And what do we have ourselves? We have a screw; such joy! Such happiness! You are as rich as a king! You ride inside like a big shot and whether it's a quick screw or something which drags on, you come out equally flaccid, shorter by a head. You can go and drip somewhere else. She, in the meantime, has climaxed at least two or three times, or more: a real devourer of prick. But that's nothing yet: she keeps some-thing from it. That's their secret: even when they don't make it, when they don't go over the top to the point of fainting, simply keeping cool, even then they can do something with it; it makes them produce and they become pregnant anyway. Whereas for us, we always have the same come-down. Forty-nine Danaids were able to use this moment to strike with a knife. It was on the way up that Achilles was struck at the heel by the arrow; hadn't heard anything, hadn't seen anything, hadn't heard anyone coming. Too far away, too busy.

It could be that woman, on the contrary, stays awake; maybe she uses her opportunity to the fullest. In the end, she's in an ideal situation. She doesn't even need, as Fredegonde did, to push him out of her bed; he's swept out through the very act. And even if he comes out of it alive, he's done for . . . ejaculate and die! Paternity is an idea. **Pater semper incertus**. *They are savage priestesses. They lie as in temple cubicles and do it with the first comer.*

All the patriarchies are a reaction against that, a jealous effort to obtain power over these bellies, to obtain authority, to stretch an arm over this progeny whose physical owner-ship one is trying to establish by any means. They go along with the game; it is called romantic love, when you are assured by word, look and gesture that you are the only one and for her the only possible one. But I could go on putting my hands on your belly, listening to the heart beats and a few days only before the birth shower the child with my semen (the Eskimos believe they feed it in that way), I could never touch it. It was a process which was taking place outside of me. If, later, we may play with him and hold him, it is through the good grace of the priestess. I saw you with Jean, with Colin, with all of them, when you didn't know I was looking at you. Looking at you, I sometimes think that that is my role in your life; to be your voyeur; because also, when we sleep together, especially then, I often have the feeling of being your onlooker; a kid who jumps after a sweet without ever catching it.

I give this lengthy confession as a document amongst others; it is the modern version of ethnographic tales of **couvade** and it expresses the same feeling. It is a kill. So then, if there

is a danger of postnatal psychosis and depression for woman,
there is equally a danger of psychosis and depression for man.

That pregnancy and the post-partum period occasion men-
tal disturbances is a clinical given, whatever opinion one
might have as to their aetiology; but that the accession to
paternity should be a problem to the extent of bringing about
serious or even minor disturbances may at first give rise to
scepticism, and if no one doubts that maternity is a major
time in the psychological evolution of woman, the study of
normal or pathological experience of paternity is curiously
neglected. (Ebtinger and Renoux, 1967).

Making a child, for one as much as for the other, does not go
without saying, for the good reason that it is the occasion for
both of them to be confronted once more with castration. But
– once more – they are not confronted at the same time, nor in
the same manner. There is discrepancy and disparity at the
level of content: it is the revelation of the loss which drives the
woman 'crazy' after the delivery. It is the faith in his products
of substitution which makes man delirious – whom I would not
necessarily call mad for all that: this is how he is more candid.
The sex change, in any case, although of a symbolic order,
cannot achieve this '**coincidentia oppositorum**' which is the
dream of the hermaphrodite.

It may be true that the life of each, man or woman, as Fliess
says, is determined by menstrual rhythms of maternal origin.
Rhythms, cycles which give woman in her body the feeling of
duration, of History. Clio is woman as Péguy already noted.
However, they must both precisely annul this belonging
which involves them very differently.

Man readily settles in eternity, even if he has a physical
rhythm. The immobility of the male system and its completely
abstract time are measured by the clock. It is probably why
one of the crucial moments of the psychotic development of
Schreber is this 'hole in time', that moment 'when the clocks
of the world have stopped'. Terre-Fleur also lives outside
of time, in his delusion. 'Time stops,' he says, 'there is no
day or night, I don't sleep. There are no meal times; I'm not
hungry.' Similarly for Robinson, who would not have aged

if the irruption of the Whitebird had not brutally slapped on him the twenty-five years of his stay on the island.

Holes in space go together with the hole in time. Aucassine says that in her delusion she would stumble into things and cross the street at any time. That is why she was hospitalized. For nothing else.

The pulse, the heart, the breathing are probably enough in each of them to provide the original model of the notch that primitive man marked in succession on the wall of his cave: $1 + 1 + 1 + 1 \ldots$ etc., for each animal killed. But if man **counts** the kills, woman is memory. She is **marked**. She knows, for example, that each mark erases the previous one and yet adds to it. She is therefore at once the ever threatening zero and the extra 1 – and thus it is inside of herself that she has the experience of the Other.

It is not possible to think, with Tournier, that the Other could be replaced with a miracle-child. As the Other, he demands to be there in the real person of a partner, and this is not in contradiction with what I have just stated about woman. For if she is not all, at least it can also be said that she is a woman and the Other. Thus she cannot do without a Father or a Husband or a Child who should be the real person of this Other according to her division. But she knows it. Passing from division to dividing, she also passes from the imaginary to the symbolic and has the experience of the desire of the Other. Love is her own experience and so is castration; for it is true, as Granoff and Périer – already quoted – say, that 'every love carries castration'.

6

Beauty

BEAUTY – Homeric attribute, as I said. Woman is beautiful by definition, since if she knows or says that she is ugly, she is no longer a woman. That is at least what is heard in analysis, where these statements do not go one without the other. And this despite the fact that, according to popular wisdom, an ugly woman is more hot-blooded than a beautiful one. Is a hot-blooded woman therefore not a woman? That is to say that a woman in our language and our society is defined by her beauty and not by her sexual capacity.

This beauty happened to provide the cinema with its raw material and if there is consuming, as one hears more than enough today, it is indeed with the eyes. Cinema consumes stars and offers them for the public's consumption. Certainly women are not alone in showing themselves on the screen. But the word 'star' is feminine and for once it is the feminine which wins out: male stars, by virtue of the phenomenon, have turned into women. That there are great films, that there are also films conceived against the very principle of the star, is not in doubt. But what drives people wild, what brings them in, is the star. To be convinced it is enough to think of the posters pinned on the cupboards of army barracks, or inside school desks. And in the street one can grab in passing the locks of Brigitte Bardot, the languishing grace of Delphine Seyrig, exhibited, provocative, as were – at one time – the bloody mouth of Joan Crawford or the pale cheek of Greta Garbo. At any rate the star did not wait for cinema in order to rule: in a century long gone, Helen's beauty was already breaking hearts; and Charmides – already a male star –

knew how to display himself. He fulfils our expectation of
a star better than Helen, he who had himself announced
everywhere, before he appeared, by the crowd's gaze turned
upon him; so that Socrates could only seize him, while expecting his appearance, as already seen, already projected,
already object of the gaze, already 'pictured' in the sense
that President Schreber understands the word (see above,
p.109).

Painting was, before cinema, the provider of shapes. Filled
with faces and flesh and breasts! And, curiously, the great
period in painting was also the time when the religious theme
ordinarily provided the content of the pictures. Avowed
eroticism has taken this place today. But there is nothing
contradictory in these displacements: there is a fine line between contemplation and consumption; even if the question
is one of **not** crossing this line; and equally between the erotic
scene and the religious scene.

The love of the udrite poets tells us what this line or this
'not' is that religion makes sacred. The love object, kept
at a distance and offering itself to contemplation, to the gaze
only, unleashes the word in the poet lover: the woman shows
herself, the poet sings. Tahar Labib Djedidi (see above, p.78),
in the work on Arab poetry already mentioned, quotes this
extract from a tale: '. . . the bride to be . . . refuses to put
back on again the shirt which she has taken off to display
herself in front of him [her fiancé] and show him that she is
without blemishes. She tells him: I shall only put it back on
if you improvise a poem.' And Tahar Labib Djedidi explains:
'The bride to be, as a woman, is defined through her body. As
for him, he must become himself in his verse.' Comparisons
with courtly poetry have not been lacking: the poet contemplates his Lady and sings of love; he does not consummate it.
'The relation beauty/chastity is striking,' notes Tahar Labib
Djedidi. 'Chastity is not a transposition of a religious feeling
here. It is not the expression of a religious continence, but that
of an excessive respect **for beauty**; the only thing is, if God is
Beauty, there is isomorphism. From the start, this relation
is incompatible with day-to-day living; to be chaste in the
presence of a (sexual) beauty, is to renounce the very symbol
of life: desire.'

Thus, **contemplating woman's beauty and not consum-mating the sexual act are one and the same thing.** It is because the love of the form is denial of the other as subject of desire. A subject who is already there, however, and insists. Only the image makes a screen against which the eye crashes without reaching the other: 'The gaze cannot reach this impenetrable woman,' says the poet. Indeed. Certainly not the gaze which distances. The gaze can penetrate nothing. The contemplated love object is always far away.

> *For you are far away*
> *my gaze comes back to me*
> *every time stretched towards you*
> *brought back through the fullness of my tears.*

This lady contemplated and never reached, is also the Only One, like the Lady of the troubadour; and the udrite poet, like the troubadour, can only die of love.

> *I swore to love only you until the time*
> *When the dust of the grave shall cover me.*

Thus beauty distances the object of man's desire; but in so doing it maintains this object in its status of object.

Similarly, her own beauty distances woman from her gaze, as the specular image already did. But since it is a question of proper beauty, the object has no longer the same status. We were able to note in passing how little consistency the object world has for woman. Words resembling those of Aucassine (see chapter 3) are frequently heard from the lips of women. Here, for example, is what Marie Cardinal writes (1973):

I had the feeling of going away, of being suddenly trans-ported far from everywhere and everything. I was nowhere. I would suddenly come back when I touched something for instance. Then the objects did not want to be touched any longer. I was as if lost in the air, like a ghost or as if dissolved; everything seemed to abandon me. I was empty, I was absent, nowhere. I was only an object. I was gone. Sometimes it was very difficult to come back because familiar objects seemed different. The air had changed and everything was foreign as if I found myself on the moon and were only an object.

One could not say better, both how objects are more than objects for woman, since they are the guarantee of her existence; and how she is for herself only an object, placed elsewhere. 'I was still very much "in" my things,' writes Mary Barnes when she tells of the fury unleashed when a friend wanted to borrow her tweezers. And she expressed the same fury if one of her paintings was moved. Her objects were truly hers in the same way as her body. Just to touch them would unleash the 'it'; it is the word she used to designate her destructive fury.

Gina Lombroso, too, speaks very well of the intimate link which binds woman to her objects; she recalls how her father, the eminent Italian criminal lawyer, having noticed that many women went mad when they were forced to move house, had proposed a law entitling them to keep their furniture in case of divorce. Lacan, on the other hand, said that woman will easily look lost: without her objects she is indeed lost. Philiberte (see above, p. 37) thinks she remembers that as a child, almost a baby, she returned with her mother to their native village, after the death of her father, and that she got desperately lost there, until the time when some local people took her back to her home which was inexplicably close. In her fright, she had probably moved away instead of staying where she was left. Now, it is said, in French, of someone who loses their mind that they 'move house' [déménagent].

Woman's relation to objects remains marked by narcissism, just as maternal love does; for the good reason that neither object nor subject are, for her, secured categories. But have we thought of what an entirely masculine world would be, full of objects, if woman was not there to return to the object its dignity of 'thing' (in Lacan's meaning)? It would very simply be full of things (in the indefinite plural).

Things with which man plays, as he already plays with his penis. I did say that the little girl does not play. At least female and male play do not have much in common. There are male games and female games; men and women analysands can say very well what game they played as children: female or male despite, in spite of, or against their sex. Jeanne, an homosexual analysand, only played boys' games with her brothers; she loved marbles and hated dolls; these days, she fixes things

around the house; climbs a ladder to repair the aerial on the
roof; takes bicycles apart and is busy with car engines. This
one plays. But the girl with her doll does not play. 'During
the Messina earthquake,' Gina Lombroso writes further,
'little girls could be seen wandering amongst the ruins defying
cold and death to find their dolls, as a mother would for
her children.' Is it not the story of Demeter all over again?
She descended into Hell to find Persephone. Demeter and
Persephone of whom Kerenyi (1967) says that they are **one**
'Double-Goddess', a major theme of femininity.

THE HOUSE AND THE IMAGE

The house is not for woman what it is for man either; because
for woman, her house is quite simply her interior; hers. She
is the keeper of the home, according to Hegel, if you wish;
but it seems to be more a phenomenon of invagination in a
seamless space.

The **house** is for woman, just as as for Descartes, Merleau-
Ponty, mystics and poets, and just as for children and the
insane, the object of objects, the '**objeu**' (a term taken from
Francis Ponge) itself [ob-game]; since it is a question of
construction and of the fact that this game results in a body
(of building, if you like). Even if it is true that it is generally
man who builds while woman decorates.

As object, the house **displays itself**. Here, for instance:
I am at my work table near the window and, if I look up, I
see a house, opposite. Thus I am at home and it is the house
opposite that I see. If I wanted to see my own house, I would
have to go out. I do not see the house I live in.

The house is therefore only an image. But, what does
it mean, the image of a house? What I see opposite is a wall,
a pile of stones. But what is a wall? A stone? Etc., etc. We
could conclude from this that we only see definitions and not
things. Better still: one never sees the whole house and it does
not even have a façade that the gaze may contain. As many
'views' as points of view. Moreover: others would have seen a
roof where I saw a house; and others 'the sky above the roof'.
And who assures me that this house is not hallucinated? On
this point, it is appropriate to reserve judgment like Freud
and Descartes, and not to pronounce oneself on the reality

of the house, and not to posit that the judgment is true: truth and reality are the two pegs of an 'inherited and completely eroded system of thought' (Lacan, 1966).

So what is it to see a house? It can be enough, in the first instance, to say: it is to pick out the object-house on the horizon, from the objects which make up its perspective, but which are not it. And if the house thus picked out is more an object than the sky, could it be that it can be of use to me? I would have chosen therefore according to a quite pragmatic interest in the **Umwelt**, as one says cleverly. However, as we noted, if I enter this house to live in it, I do not see it. In order to see it, I am forced to remain at a distance. To see a house is therefore to live in it as little as possible. It remains to conclude that if I see the house, it is because I want to see it, quite simply. In other words: because it is the most pregnant form of my desire, the one that is most full of desire.

Starting from there, but from there only, it has its own life, of separate form in which we wish to believe. As a seen object, as a form, it can be photographed or projected on a screen. It then becomes fascinating and nails me to the spot. At the right **distance**. It is the specular material of the visual arts. That is why one should not confuse what is seen on the screen for the pleasure of seeing, and what is seen in the street for everyday needs; but one may also enjoy looking at those same objects in the street which are of some use in other ways. There is a specular quality in every object as a constituent of the object; but, on the other hand, it is quite true that I need this house to have a reality.

It is appropriate here to go again through the detour of the mirror stage (Lacan, 1966). For in it we see the opening of the hiatus which distances the image from the subject: symmetrical and reversed image which the mother already knew, which the desire of the mother already isolated from the background [**fond**: both 'background' and 'content'] against which the child was moving. This is what makes the content and the form, and not a structure inherent to the object. And such is the function of the beloved double: intangible, it formalizes; if I touch it, it vanishes like an apparition. If I concretize it – build it in solid – it becomes an object and lasts for ever; but equally, as rubbish, it is fated to destruction. And so it is for every body forcibly cut from me. If I know that the house is

my double, my face projected at a distance, the same and an
other that I saw once in a mirror, I also know that at every
moment, I must make it appear – but equally seize it as form
of the desire of the other. The house then gains in reality and
beauty and, although ephemeral, it becomes eternal; what
is more moving than the struggle of beauty and death on a
face?

In order for me to see my face in the mirror and the house in
the sky, it is necessary and it is enough that by accident they
happened to be the form of the **desire of an other**. Otherwise
there is no mirror, and consequently no face; and no sky,
and consequently no house. It is necessary for it indeed –
mirror or sky – that there be a screen woven from the point
of crossing (or mesh) between two desires. It is there, at this
crossing, that the little reality of objects and their beauty
hang; I am deluded if I believe that this form is me or someone
or something. From narcissistic delusion to joy, there is only
this little reality.

To sum up:

1. The house is at a distance. Seeing it is living in it as little as
possible. It is to not live in it. It is then seen in the space that
perhaps it organizes and orientates.

2. Inside, from where I can come out, since I can come in,
it is empty like the mustard pot or the word of the Lacanian
potter. It is a cocoon with a door.

3. It is an object concerning the scopic drive. As such, the
house comes after the specular image and after the image
of the mother (not historically, however). The substitution
of one image for another clearly indicates that they already
belong to the register of the symbolic. (cf. Winnicott's tran-
sitional object whose essential point is the dynamic of substitution that it implies.)

4. It is constructed like an 'objeu', going from the cliché to
the most inexpressible form of desire or to the simple dream,
like Jean-Jacques Rousseau's house with green shutters.

From then on, questions multiply: **sight** has a decisive
function in the libidinal economy, a function which institutes,
constitutes the object of the gaze in its reality **of object**. It is
not a statement of the obvious; the image is not a pure fantasy

inasmuch as it is the image of the Other, that the Other sees and that the Other reflects. Sight would then be situated in the area of **sublimation**, since sublimation marks the moment of socialization of the libido and it is a component drive which would decide on sublimation.

There is colour and – **a contrario** – the grey world of schizophrenics and the black of Mary Barnes. Now, colour is space, the 'invariable of space', as Michel Serres writes. Black, when it is negation of colour, if that is the case, would then be the void. As for grey, 'whoever has once mixed colours knows that if he despairs of finding the right tone, the appropriate nuance of blue or green, greyness threatens: this mobile dirt on the palette which merges everything and cancels everything and which cannot even be erased because erasing is greyness itself', writes the psychoanalyst Pierre Beaudry. And, he concludes, '"greyness" is therefore neither a colour, nor a non-colour, but the "almost", the "quasi", the "not quite" of the generalized defection in the lack of seeing.'

But it is beauty which is in question here. Is there a step to take between the specular image and the beautiful? And from the beautiful to the one, or from the one to the beautiful? The ugly is not watchable. Neither is the infinite; nor the multiple, nor even two objects. But the one will not let itself be stared at. Where then can we arrest and rest our gaze? On the body? It has been said that it is 'absolute body' when it becomes an object of contemplation (Maillet, 1974): it seems that it needs to evacuate its organic complexity, its expanse and its alterations and also its thickness, in order to become specular material. Its relation to the face does not go without saying either. Isn't the face more **one** than the body? And the eyes more so than the face? And the gaze itself, more so than the eyes? But then who is watching what? Leonardo could not find the face of Christ for the *Last Supper*. A hole in the place of the face. Nicolas de Staël always paints at the limit of the hole; he opens the way for our gaze on to an object in space, an object which was not there a moment earlier; and it is there as if on the first day. Born as if out of effraction, at the limit of the visible and the invisible: it is the subject of what Merleau-Ponty writes and what de Staël paints, at the same period.

If sight has a determining function, so then has the component character of the drive; for the subject reaches a little
reality only in the effraction, through using one function instead of another and inverting the objects of each: the scopic
drive instead of the anal drive; an object to see instead of an
object to leave. If a drive could be complete, it would reach
its end – satisfaction – and it would miss its aim, in the event
aesthetic pleasure (cf. the trajectory of the drive, above, pp.
70–1). Art is therefore absolutely necessary. 'The picture
world is a wall, but all the birds in the sky may fly in it freely
. . . at every depth,' writes de Staël. The painter flattens the
objects to create depth. The picture wall is not there as a plug,
but in order to offer to the gaze something other than the
black hole of the invisible, devoid of meaning, on the one
hand; and, on the other, something other than the ready-
made world of daily life or of science.

Sublimation could be defined in this context, as Lacan does
when he writes: 'Sublimation raises the object to the dignity
of the Thing', and 'anamorphosis is a kind of construction
made in such a way that through an optical transposition, a
certain shape which at first is not perceptible emerges from
what is to begin with indecipherable' (Lacan, 1973). It is
exactly the definition of the specular image (and that of the
object-house) as optical construction in space; and it is that
of every object.

Form, therefore, constructs. But it constructs in solid,
as I have said; because it constructs in the real, even if the
world, in relation to the squalid, seems to be only an image.
And even if the beauty of the body is not in the body, it is
inscribed in the real; and sublimation must not be understood
as dematerialization. Similarly, the troubadour's contemplation does not turn his Lady into an ethereal creature, nor
does it make him impotent. I happened to hear one day, on
the radio, these unforgettable verses by an Arab poet:

When you walk on my grave
I shall tear my shroud with desire.

It is sexual desire which is in question. Djedidi repeats it
insistently: beauty provokes sexual desire while forbidding
it, since it is intangible. But the eye has no other place to rest.

It wanders a long time; Musil says that 'finding the beautiful is first of all finding'. But once the object of the gaze has been found, the gaze can no longer look anywhere else. Any woman, anybody cannot bring forth the beautiful image for a subject. What is needed is the encounter of two **subjects**. Pygmalion was in love with his statue, and today the story of 'Monsieur Klebs et Rosalie' (Obaldia, 1975) tells the same love. But that is a fantasy and a very male one, which reduces a woman to a mass of rubber or a piece of marble; whereas woman turns the smallest piece of cloth into flesh. As far as sublimation is concerned, it arises only between flesh and flesh; subject and subject. The Only One is the one in the encounter which is at once the most unexpected and the most necessary: love at first sight.

That a woman may be the only one for a man, as the poets wished, turns this woman into the absolute object, in the same way that she is the 'absolute body', an idolatrous myth where the subject itself plunges; one might as well choose the mystic path. But equally the woman who turns a man into the Only One is a mystic.

The double
She at least gets something out of turning man into the Only One, for her image is now seen and recognized by someone. She no longer needs to believe in it. What a relief. Man, on the contrary, experiences no relief in being for a woman the face of faces; he is not an image; he does not have a 'face' [**figure**: both 'face' and 'representation']. Woman does not represent him in plastic works as man has always done with her. And he himself does not normally turn his image into a more virulent double. In the cases of male psychosis, the double is as persecutory as it can be for a woman; but I doubt that one could find in men a case as perfect and exemplary (inasfar as every woman may recognize herself in it) as that of an analysand called Bob: a young woman with a masculine morphology and a masculine name. Her original woman's name is Lucette. But no one calls her Lucette, neither her husband, nor even her parents. Lucette is only the name of her persecutory double. Lucette calls out to Bob incessantly and violently. She insults him and reproaches him for everything she is, to the extent of

driving him to the brink of suicide. Who then is Lucette? Her
double or herself? And Bob? (Rank, 1932).

Such is the object for woman, at first: her **double**, her specular image. Every object retains something of this status, and she is for herself an object. Thus she is forced to perfect it (herself), inasmuch as it does not fulfil its function – which it never does – of complement in the edification of the unity of the subject. Woman is here a Pygmalion for herself, and I called Pygmalion the twenty-five year old woman, married and mother of a little boy, whose only passion was to remake herself. A small clerk, she had managed to find the ways and the means to have her nose and her chin remodelled. But she could already foresee that wrinkles would come. She decided then to prevent them and to return to a clinic for her eyelids and her neck – which she did. But she did not stop there. A few years later, she did not have an inch of cartilage, nor even a square of original skin, I dare say. That is when she left husband and child (she had always beaten the child; and she had already left the husband, not for a lover, but for herself); she went abroad with her new face. She probably hoped to begin again incognito somewhere else. She went mad there, was locked up in a psychiatric hospital and then was brought back to France. Women's relentlessness in 'making themselves a face', as they say, is equalled only by their relentlessness in cleaning or tidying. It has to hold together; it must be pleasing to look at. If it does not stand up; if it is not pleasing to look at, it is because the ever threatening gap between her and her doubles is opening up; and beyond; the void.

The detachable object
It is this faultless image which circulates amongst men and used to circulate as object of exchange in primitive societies.

Man's penis has never been put in circulation nor has man himself. They are not objects of exchange. The penis can only be stolen in the manner of the 'flying penis' mentioned above, which can be stolen since it flies [**voler**: both 'to steal' and 'to fly']: but precisely, in that dream, the penis becomes a separate object for the female imaginary – which it is not – and woman can, henceforth, incorporate it. 'She imagines, from then on, that this penis belongs to her,' writes Lilian Rotter (1932), 'and she feels entitled to consider this part of the external world as something belonging to her Ego.' That is the whole difference between a man and a woman: the penis is not detachable.

On the contrary, what is detached from the body of woman, faeces, periods, or child, is part of her being. As for her breasts; they are not amongst the objects she loses; that is why they can be the equivalent of the penis. Thanks to this game of substitution between objects, detachable or not, penis envy could perhaps develop, according to Lilian Rotter's argument – the penis that woman experiences as hers at the time of coitus.

On the contrary for man, this **non-detachable** object, the penis, is **figurable**. It is on this model that his object world and artistic universe are constructed. The curious thing is that, passing into the register of the constructed or the represented, the primarily non-detachable object acquires an autonomy which the object of female drives never has. But it can be understood, since this penis of which man is in fear of being deprived is, however, never **identifiable** with the body, nor with half the body: a castrated man never loses his life, as we see in Dominique Fernandez's *Porporino* (1974). And he even acquires singing in the process. The stakes, once again, are not the same.

Man can therefore figure his penis; he can also play with it, or use it, or enjoy it, or arm himself with it; but he never becomes confused with the object (except in pathological cases). Woman comes naturally to take for him that place of object which she already is for herself. And man, then, plays with her, or enjoys her, or adorns himself with her as with the phallus.

I will be told that I am behind and that the woman-object is over. She no longer wants this status. Yes: but this wanting must still fit in at that point where the scopic drive takes over from anality. In woman, the part of herself which falls if it is not held, the deciduous part, is the child **par excellence**. But she never recognizes the child as a foreign body. On the model of this primary object (not in time, of course), every object still pertains to woman, after separation. On the other

what she loses. As reaching the genital drive does not hold for
woman the decisive feature that it does for man, she remains
governed – as we noted – by the scopic drive; for longer and
more essentially. And the danger remains that she may close
herself up in a narcissistic structure.

MARY BARNES

Hence woman's difficulty in creating, even as a painter. The
example of Mary Barnes (1971) shows how the passage comes
about. It is with her shit (literally) that she draws her first
breasts or signs [**seins** or **signes**] on the wall of her room, in
Kingsley Hall. But previously, she had already been mould-
ing and sculpting it. She talked one day of 'a sculpture, not
alive, yet **complete** in itself, fully satisfying'. It is therefore a
question of giving the anal object its status of object one, even
if it should be inanimate. 'Amongst all those whom I heard
speak, not one comes to the point of distinguishing the thing
which, separate from all others, makes art,' says Heraclitus
(quoted by Ramnoux, 1974).

In her approximately annual descents into madness, between 1965 and 1970, Mary Barnes sinks into her shit. Then
she stops eating; she cannot get out of bed: 'in bed going inside
myself for the second time'. She is under a black blanket.
The walls are black. It is a grave and she falls into it. She
comes out of it **thanks** to her anality; she enjoys transforming
her excrements into visible signs 'as pure as Zen characters',
notes her therapist, Joe Berke. Rezvani (1976) does not speak
any differently of the 'trace', the 'stamp' that the painter
marks out in space, and he immediately evokes 'the gesture of
the child who generously offers his excrements to the Other,
smearing everything he touches (signing it, leaving the print
of his many fingers on the walls) like the first man-painter
marking with his print the wall of the cave-belly'.

Mary no longer covers herself with her excrements, no
longer hides in them, loses herself in them, nor gets merged
with them. She enjoys seeing them, and in the enthusiasm
of her discovery, she spills all over Kingsley Hall. The whole
community has to love her stinking frescoes; otherwise she is
not loved. If she is not loved, it is because she is wicked and

must be punished. Then, all that is left is to destroy things and people and herself. It is the 'it' which explodes. Her bomb.

But Joe Berke loves her paintings. He loves Mary; he bathes her without repulsion, it seems, when she is covered in shit and he is so strong that she cannot destroy him; she cannot hurt him. Therefore she is good and has the right to live and to paint.

The yearly relapses were provoked by the difficulty the members of the community experienced in putting up with her spilling out and her violence; they could no longer tolerate the 'monster of Kingsley Hall'. It wasn't enough for Mary that her 'inside' became her 'outside', according to the phrase which heads this chapter. It had to be outside properly speaking, that is to say for others to look at. It is at this point of no return – for, in spite of the relapses, there was no longer simple repetition – that the handling of Mary's transference by Joe Berke played a decisive role. And it is at this point that scopic sublimation plays its role.

There was another path for Mary: faith. She herself compares her 'downs', her 'ups', her 'night' and her resurrection to the mystical steps of St John of the Cross. Faith and madness [**foi** and **folie**] are almost the same word. 'My faith and my madness are the two great events of my life. Madness brought out and revealed the faith that was in me. Going through madness is a purification which brings me closer to God, helps me to understand Him better and to penetrate more completely into His **vision**' (my emphasis). She identifies with Christ as she does with Berke. On the other hand, her faith goes through her painting. She starts painting crucifixions and resurrections.

Here is the account Joe Berke gives of a painting session:

I recall one occasion, early one afternoon, when I walked into the Games Room just as she was about to begin a painting. She had nailed large sheets of white paper, maybe eight feet high by twelve feet long, on the wall facing the dining-room. Without so much as making a preliminary drawing, Mary took up a brush, dipped it in one of several buckets, and sloshed away at the wall. Within minutes, vigorous yet delicate dashes of colour covered an area **several times the size of Mary.** *Then she picked up a smaller brush and started to fill in the characters. Never once did she stop or look up although, as she worked, she would often laugh, or talk or even scream at this or that figure (or vice versa – she played all parts), as the figure began to make his presence known in the painting. From time to time a beautiful smile would break across her face. It was as if, at that moment, she had transcended all her troubles and entered an ecstatic reverie.*

Leon came in, then others. Mary did not notice. She was totally engrossed in her work, in herself. No one spoke, only an infrequent gasp or cough interrupted the drama that was unfolding across our wall. From time to time Leon would point to this or that figure and I, or someone else, would nod, or smile, or perhaps just look on, too enchanted to reply.

One hour passed, two hours, then Mary stepped back from the burst of colour lying resplendent in front of us and sank to the ground, exhausted. She had brought to life the transfiguration *of Christ.* (my emphasis)

It is indeed a question of transfiguration, and more specific-ally of the passage to figuration. Colours now give the solidity of space to signs. From then on there is a change of object. The mother is finally displaced. There is an inside and an outside, a subject and an other, a subject and objects. She can even allow herself to love her mother. At last, the 'separation' (it is the very term used by Joe Berke) occurs, has occurred, when Mary goes out for her one weekly psychotherapy session at Joe Berke's – instead of waiting for him at Kingsley Hall. Separation in and of space, separation in and of time.

Phallic beauty
The separate body – the body thus separated – is already governed by the phallic function. Standing up, instead of staying in bed, going up and coming up again: it is the phallic function which is at work. It is that function which ensures that the body doesn't crumble into dust, doesn't rot away, doesn't dissolve into the night, but remains whole and one, and visible: like the sculpted turd of Mary. It is less the love

of life than the love of that which stands up and holds us and which, by this fact, appears.

The **phallic** function is specifically that which also ensures that the penis becomes **erect**. Then it becomes flaccid again: it goes down. These are not metaphors. How is it that this spectacular penis, thus erected, doesn't ordinarily become object of pleasure for itself, but is the instrument of sexual enjoyment? And that it finds its pleasure in penetrating another body? And how is it that the object of love and contemplation, namely beauty, the cause of love at first, slides and gives its place to the object (a)?

Man is not fascinated by the image, as we said, and his object relation is different. The 'separation' has occurred from the time of the constitution of the specular image. But, however captive of this image woman remains, she cannot find her **jouissance** in fascination either. Inasfar as she remains captive of her beauty, she also remains frigid and passive. . . Passive since fascinated, indeed; staggered and staggering.

This beauty – a sign that matter no longer falls – is, however, moving only in a real matter and a real body. This being true for both man and woman. Man, just as woman, sees at first. And for both, beauty is the beauty of the body. The sign, of course, is neither objectively founded, nor universal: to each his own. Ten-cents beauty or rare beauty, each has their beauty for someone; even a monster: the child is beautiful; the adolescent is beautiful; the girl is beautiful; the woman is beautiful. The difference is to be found in that man is the one who looks rather than sees. And woman sees rather than looks. She even has visions, as has been said.

And that is why Philiberte was homosexual – or hommo-sexual. Inexhaustible when she speaks of beauty, Philiberte tells us:

As a little girl, I loved beauty passionately. But I knew that I didn't really love beautiful children or beautiful girl friends; only their beauty. It was a matter of indifference to me to leave them over the summer holidays. I would take some photos and they would be enough. I would question the photos at length. . .

. . . Sometimes, when my girl friend was in front of me, I 143
would mentally look at her photo; and even, at times, to see BEAUTY
it I had to turn around; her real presence disturbed me.

And again:

*Because of my indifference, because of what everyone used
to call my coolness, it hadn't occurred to me that I was
homosexual. And yet, I already liked stroking those faces:
they moved me; I thought it was enough for me to recognize
them with the tip of my fingers; to see them with my fingers.
But where to stop?*

 *I keep on thinking that I didn't love this woman who made
me cross the line of homosexuality and when I didn't find her
beautiful, I would find her ugly.*

Oscillation where castration is verified: 'When I didn't find
her beautiful, I would find her ugly.' What does that mean?
The ugly is not the opposite of the beautiful, however. The
ugly is the deformed, not the shapeless; the horrible, not the
black. It is still something that is seen and not the invisible.
It appears just as the beautiful does. Only, it is not cause of
love. It violates the gaze of the subject who sees, although if the
latter sees, it is the sign that he looks at, which is somewhat in
connivance. To see and to look, at once call upon each other
and cancel each other out. The subject who shows himself
ugly violates the gaze. And what he shows is his need and
not his desire; for need is without law or castration, through
which it destroys desire. Inasfar as desire is the principle
of the subject, the subject who shows himself ugly is himself
destroyed.

 But indeed, the ugly through laying bare the need has
a function. 'Whoever wants to become an angel, becomes a
beast'; the woman who wants to be beautiful, and condemns
her lover to contemplation, becomes a beast and only shows a
grimace. The beast with its needs, its hunger, its warts, shows
through, destroying the beloved form. Devouring and no
longer contemplating. But is it not the same drive reversed?
The ugly is of the same register as the beautiful and the aesthetic experience is sustained only through their oscillation.

 The opposite of the beautiful would be rather the night and,
in the experience of the beautiful, the hole which appears

in place of the face. Thus beauty cannot be proposed as an ideal. The cause of love, it forbids it, if it also wishes to be its object and its aim. That is how it involves castration. Thus the painter gives up making the portrait of the Only One, as Leonardo gave up finding the face of Christ. The admission of impotence by Rezvani (see above, p. 139), condemning 'th cannibal art' of the hero of *Le portrait ovale*, reiterates in an exemplary fashion the failure of the painter confronted with any object, as well as with a woman or his beloved woman.

Inasfar as man looks at, then contemplates, woman, she is for him, as for herself – rather than fantasy or object (a) – the big O barred (Ø): the thing barred through its lack. But if she is not the object (a), beauty is fatally cashed in on.

To say therefore that beauty is (Ø) and not (A), nor (a), is to say that it is constitutive of the object for a subject, to the extent – as we shall see – of the Other resisting as subject.

Object and nothing else than object, that is to say: nothing, up to this point. And not the Other. Nothing if not for the fact – and there lies the paradox – that there is beauty only in another subject. Thus it is as S (Ø) that beauty is cause of love; for it reveals to a subject the proximity of the object as subject, an imminent revelation which, in the sexual act, provokes **jouissance**.

From which it follows that there is beauty only in human-kind. Admiring the animals drawn by Frédéric Rossif for a television programme – drawn indeed – I tell myself that they probably move me because the gaze of a man addresses their astonishing beauty to me and that it is this that my gaze meets. But also because the perfect animal movement is already, for this dancer that is man – and for him exclusively –, dance. My eye (or Frédéric Rossif's) follows the spine of the beast, up to the neck, the muzzle and seeks the gaze. The animal's gaze is deeply moving in that it is opaque and at the same time ver-tiginous. Is it because pure desire inhabits this body without subject? Or need? Rather need. But man is a being of desire. Need horrifies him, he disguises animal need into desire and he turns the expression of human need into a fantasy.

The animal doesn't look at me as I look at it. It expects signals, not words; and our words as well as our gaze are only signals for it.

A fortiori beautiful things; they are so only through the effect of our anthropomorphism; for they do not look at us. The beauty or the ugliness of things or beasts are thus the emergence of our fantasies and of our phobias. So-called female fantasy: the cat; male fantasy: the horse or the dog; both objects, upon which the phobia of the opposite sex is crystallized. Penis-snake; penis-fish; sacred cow; spider of the sex; insects, Medusas and various monsters, this whole arsenal is reduced to the beautiful (or ugly) object which, already a monster, displays the object of desire as if it were there. The same beauty as that which, attributed to woman, turns her into a beast and, attributed to the beast, turns her into a woman, as we see through *The Story of O* (Réage, 1954).

It is thus as animal beauty that woman is the fantasy of man. But human beauty is something quite else. I remember having seen a photograph of Brigitte Bardot on all fours in front of a kennel. We know for certain that Brigitte Bardot is not a bitch, and **that is why** this image moves us, even though it has been conceived to feed male fantasies – as well as female fantasies.

But neither fantasized beauty nor fantasized ugliness are the sex proper. 'The sex covers itself, out of modesty,' says Nasio, and again: 'The fear of the Medusa head doesn't originate in the analogy with the hairy sex of woman. The sex is not traumatic. The representation of the Medusa was needed for it to become so. Trauma comes only after the event' (Nasio and Taillandier, unpublished). Indeed, neither a piece of flesh, nor a hole of flesh are beautiful, ugly or horrible. What the gaze turns away from is the figure of castration. This figure is composed by the subject's gaze. He does not create it out of nothing; but out of the agency of need in the other. Such a need always finds its object in a victim which offers itself because it already is a victim in its own fantasy: death by tearing, devouring or engulfing. The threat is directed at the sex, already a wound, and carries death. $\mathcal{S} \lozenge a$, this formula of fantasy where, as Lacan says, 'the subject fades in front of the object of desire', clearly shows that the object of the fantasized desire is a nothingness into which the subject rushes and disappears. On the contrary, beauty leaves the subject at a distance; we could say it therefore also leaves him a chance.

But if it nails him to the spot, even at the right distance; if it staggers him, if it petrifies him, it becomes a fantasy once more. But who is looking then? Beauty looks at itself; but does it look? It is paradoxical to suppose that it has a gaze; the least experience in the matter reveals that there is beauty only when it is both caught and contemplated. It would seem consequently that it is looked at but doesn't look. **In truth, either there is a subject on both sides; or there is no subject on either side.** When there is only a gaze left, the looking subject sinks; the object of the gaze becomes a monstrous thing showing itself; it is no longer Beauty, but the petrifying gaze of the Medusa. A single phobic gaze because the object then is looking. The bar of Ø expresses this paradox: it says that the object of the gaze is barred by its lack; a lack which is precisely the mark of the subject. The female sham consists in the woman knowing she is looked at but leading people to believe that she doesn't know it; however it is not properly speaking a sham, since woman doesn't look. The abuse, in this game of drives as in any other, is rather the fact of the man looking and being assured of his gaze: as if the distribution of a looking subject and a looked-at object went without saying.

The **gaze** of man, which is defined as reducing the world to objects, needs rather to be deposed as gaze. The woman is divided: she looks at man, but has the faculty of **seeing** herself and so runs the risk of objectifying herself; but if she gives this up, she deprives herself also of any symbolic opening. There is neither symmetry nor meeting between both gazes, but rather a triangulation, which could be represented as follows.

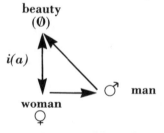

Thus the most inextricable ambiguity necessarily muddles this policy which aims at giving the gaze back to woman, the right to look [**droit de regard**: 'the right to control']. As though she didn't have it! This policy probably means only that woman no longer intends to be beauty or Medusa for man's gaze. But why would man and woman have the same gaze, since they do not have the same sex? This same gaze piercing the world through and through would ruin the symbolic order.

In fact woman doesn't look; she displays herself; she is beauty. Being beauty, she is also object of love, in the same way as the beautiful adolescents of Socrates. But as the reference itself proves, it is a question of a place that woman may occupy or not, and so may man or not: that of lover. The same reference tells us that for Socrates every adolescent was like a white plumb-line on a white wall, that is to say indistinctly beautiful. Similarly, woman for the man who loves all women, is proof that the (a) gains the advantage again, as cause of desire, in place of the (Ø), cause of love. When (a) and (Ø) coincide, it is the 'burning desire' which inflames both man and woman, and Socrates as well at the sight of Charmides upon whom he doesn't rush, although he feels like putting his hand up his shirt, but whom, on the contrary, having recovered his composure after such turmoil, he questions at length.

When beauty is only (O) unbarred, whole object and not subject, it makes (O) and $ ◇ a coincide: it is the adventure of O, sacrificed on the altar of some god, and it is the story of Bellezza, the sister of the Amazon; Bellezza having no voice, it is the Amazon who speaks.

STOLEN BEAUTY

Coming from a princely family on her mother's side and from a northern upper-class family on her father's side – a cavalry officer, moreover – the Amazon scared men and women as soon as she appeared in a psychodrama group: six foot, a regal carriage, the ease of a model, the voice of a man, with a frankly scabrous language; women shrivelled and men looked down. And yet it wasn't she – the second of four daughters – who was the beauty of the family. But without question, the eldest; renamed Bellezza as soon as she was born, soon mesmerizing family and friends, to the extent that everybody around her was called: Bellezza's parents, Bellezza's sisters, Bellezza's cousins, etc.

This is how the Amazon tells the story:

'Beautiful, yes she was. My father would have liked me to be as beautiful. But she was stupid, absolutely stupid.'

'Stupid? How?' we asked.

'Well, she couldn't learn anything . . . she never learned how to ride for instance. Whereas I. . .'

And she went on to confess that her great remorse was that her father, who had come back from the war gassed and suffering from tuberculosis, died after giving her one last riding lesson that she had practically demanded.

'Yes I was an excellent rider, and I could keep a man. My sister became a whore.'

Bellezza got divorced and was unable to keep her children. The Amazon's husband was sent by the family to collect her, on the other side of the world.

'He wasn't coming back. He was made a prisoner. I know I had sent him there. I've always passed my men on to my sister. But then I got scared.'

The Amazon would pass her men to Bellezza. But apparently not for her to keep them.

'Or else had she understood at last?'

'He finally came back, after three months. So did she. She sleeps around. She's not so beautiful any more. In the end, I'm more beautiful than her. I've taken her place.'

The epilogue, in the group, is worth telling. A young woman, whom we shall call Mimosas, ventures to confess that she is frightened of the Amazon. To which the latter replies that this Mimosas has really been getting on her nerves for a long time. Mimosas starts crying right away, and says that the Amazon is 'just like her own sister, such a feminine seducer who excluded her, who always took everything from her'.

Everything, that is to say her mother and her grandmother; for her father was 'for her', the eldest who had a career like the Amazon. But in front of the Amazon, Mimosas is as though in front of an eldest and she cries like a younger one, thereby reversing the roles. And Mimosas even calls on the woman therapist, as she used to call on her mother, begging her to acknowledge the wickedness of the Amazon and her own weakness.

From then on, we no longer know who is the beauty, who

is the girl-woman and who is the girl-boy; who is the youngest
and who is the eldest. Who is the parent that one 'keeps to
oneself', the father or the mother. Things become even more
complicated when Mimosas chooses – at random – a shy
newcomer, who turns out to be the elder sister of a younger
one, a 'seducer' whom she hates.

If one thinks that this session was following another where
there had been talk of an 'awful brooch' that their mothers
gave their respective daughters as a birthday present – a
brooch which they refused and promptly lost – and that one
of these daughters was actually Mimosas, it becomes clear
that beauty is this jewel that the mother has given or not
instead of something else (the female sex). The daughters who
were not provided for had to seek comfort with their father
with whom they then identified, and like a man, they had a
career.

But femininity remained alongside beauty, imaginarily,
with the other. The loss is irreparable and they cry; unless
they go on fighting like the Amazon, who covers herself with
enormous spiky rings and wild necklaces, and makes herself
up like an idol. 'It amuses me to scare people,' she says in her
slow and noble baritone, which bursts out like thunder in its
sudden force. And the group keeps quiet.

A story of women, therefore, where man appears only at
the periphery, like a penis to get instead of the declined gift;
while the love object remains the mother; where the longed-
for gift is the gift from the mother; in the shape of beauty and
femininity.

A mirror story where the eldest is always also potentially
the youngest for another; beauty is the attribute of another,
like femininity; and the gift is what the other has received.

However stolen they may be, these attributes are frightening, and it is the fear of the phallic woman: powerful, dangerous, crushing, murderous: the Amazon. The fear is always the
same fear; it is always the fear of our 'infantile' and 'primitive'
ancestors.

The aggressive beauty of the Amazon is only the effect
of an appropriation and even of a theft: she stole her sister's
beauty, from her sister; on her face is superimposed another
face; it is a double mask, and the doubling up denounces the

mechanism of the exclusive demand for the gaze. In that sense the Amazon's beauty is only the product of her demand and not the cause of the love of the other.

The function of beauty as a mask is perfectly illustrated in a case presented by William G. Niedermann (1975). As one could expect, it is the case of a woman. From the start, she announces to her therapist that she has a facial scar; then she will not mention it for a long time. Even though the therapist keeps scrutinizing her face, he sees nothing. It is because since the age of nine, at her mother's instigation, the young woman has learned how to make herself up so as to hide completely what looks like a bruise. Did her mother not send her cowering in the bathroom when there were visitors? This thing to hide was indeed well hidden. But this is how the young woman later (the analysis lasted seven years) described this 'birthmark' [in English in the original]. 'It is a web of veins, of reddish, pinkish, bluish fibres; of discoloured flesh and skin, often hot and beating like a pulse.' The analyst notes that one sees surfacing in this description the 'unconscious equation' between the Medusa head and the scar: quite exactly the awful turquoise that her mother gave Mimosas. But the misfortune of this patient is not to be able to reject the jewel. She has a passion for precious stones, which she collects for their 'purity', whereas her own flesh is impure: since according to her the facial wound contaminates the whole person. She spends several hours every day in front of her mirror and when things don't go her way, she breaks everything; violence and depression alternate. She has the same passion for dressing and for arranging and decorating for ever new flats; she is primarily concerned with lighting and the play of colours. The result is always disappointing. So she sells and starts again somewhere else.

It is the mother obviously who gave her this awful face and this hateful female sex. And the young woman asks the therapist to magically rebirth her with a new face. Her face will not change but she will become a poet.

Niedermann explains the symmetrical faces and the over-perfect bodies of the painter David through this same reparative wish. He discovered that in fact David had an ugly scar on his upper lip. Men are not safeguarded, quite obviously, against what he calls 'facial disfigurement' [in English in the

original]: it is a question, as Niedermann says in conclusion,
of saving face. For 'the only beauty is that of the face'.

It is also a question, while saving face, of hiding the sex, as
previously, with the asexual specular image.

The Amazon was hiding her sex under the make up. But if
beauty has the reparative function of a mask, it lacks what
specifies it as a useless and vain object, which would be and
could be nothing else but a cause of love.

The example which follows Niedermann's article (Mintz,
1975) is the very demonstration of the metaphorical signification of the stain. It is about a six-year-old male child
afflicted with a grave eczema. This child would ask his mother
when she was in her bath to open the door so that he could
show her his 'pusticles'. The therapist immediately associated
'pusticles' and 'testicles' [in English in the original]. There
was indeed a very strong erotic bond between the child and
the mother, who was neglected by an impotent father. The
intention of the child was of course to show his naked mother
something in place of his own sex; but also, showing his own
sex, to see his mother's. Apart from the fact that one can draw
from this exemplary story the whole meaning of the popular
expression **'aller se faire voir'** ['get lost'; lit. 'go and show
yourself'], it effects a taking apart of the function of the gaze
by the very fact that this function unfolds here in various
stages: bringing a metaphorical object in place of the sex and
displaying instead of looking. Thus, who looks at whom and
at what? No one can say.

Is beauty as a mask only that as well: what is shown in place
of the sex? An analysand told me that she had provoked a
crisis in her psychopathic son, normally calm and respectful,
in appearing in front of him one evening, dressed (or rather
undressed) to go out for dinner with some friends. What
appeared to the boy was not his mother's beauty, his mother's
face, but her nakedness, her sex. The thing without a gaze
was thrown in his face outside of any symbolic mediation,
blocking him as subject capable of love. Without mediation,
I said (the O is not barred there); and therefore without
left-over. This everything-goes precipitates the subject into
the bottomless hole of the single gaze. It remains that the

contemplation of beauty – even if it is not reduced to its function of mask – no more implies encounter or harmony. If there is no sexual relation, there is no relation of contemplation either; even though man and woman live daily on beauty as they do on sex. Beauty is the ultimate veil which reveals the presence of the Other, beyond which limit there is nothing else than a sex without subject, whereas within there is no one yet.

CONCLUSION

Woman is the figure of this scene of the veil which covers over the primal scene: she dances the eternal and often ridiculous dance of the veil. She is alone in knowing what nothingness it is intended to veil, while man, fascinated, looks on. Thanks to which, the sexual act can take place.

Successful copulation and orgasm are certainly not the aim of the analytic treatment. However, it happens that they may, in addition, signal its outcome. Or at least it can be said that man and woman have no better opportunity than sexual relation to settle their difficult allegiance to castration, which is the experience for each that their desire is the desire of the Other. Here again, I shall quote Myriam Pécaut (1974-5): 'Healed by God, after the divine operation, the wound was to leave no visible trace in man's side; henceforward, nothing prevented him from repressing this wound elsewhere, towards woman, in other words **symbolizing** it by making it or calling it woman.' And I would add: the temptation was great for woman to heal her always reopened wound, through **symbolizing** in man the remedy, the miracle-phallus, the doctor-god.

If she doesn't see a penis when she looks at her sex, if she only sees a hole there, it's all profit, since she is not called upon to build mountains on this penis or any other! Why want to see, when there is nothing real to see in one or the other? The feminine claim here – I mean for those who ask that their own gaze be given back to them – gets carried away in an illusory project. It is, on the contrary, in difference that woman may still find herself, resisting man's prestige, to the extent of not wanting this prestige, this right to control, this power to reduce the world to objects. At the price of this resistance, a word may fall, not from one rather than the other, but between the two.

But, to take up a term that Hélène Cixous is fond of (cf. above, p. 61) what will then be woman's 'own'? Ownership is, indeed, what has been in question since the beginning of history. So far, man has managed to buy or exchange women at the pro rata of their beauty. What other combination are we proposed? The worst would be that of a double and respective appropriation; woman, for her part, appropriating an 'endless and aimless body, without main bits . . . immense astral space'; the body of the mother, in other words. Yet another way of going round castration.

Now, the wound on man's side is still there and if woman is this wound, then it is because she is his truth, as she is his beauty. 'Do not uncover the nakedness of your father's wife, it is the nakedness of your father.' It is a prescription drawn from Leviticus by Myriam Pécaut, who comments thus: 'That which is uncovered with the nakedness is a gap or a flaw'; but in truth, man is as naked as woman.

That beauty as ornament, that is to say as weapon and as cover, hides the unbearable nakedness, that is its most common function. Henceforward, it serves as any (a). In its function of Ø, on the other hand, it ensures the opening of the signifying chains, for the caesura of the subject and the object, and it is the cause of love.

If there is only one word for calling man and woman and for distinguishing them from animals – which are not naked and neither are they dressed – and if that word is precisely **man**, this comes about through a deliberate denunciation, on the part of woman, of her own body, in favour of beauty – through which man also finds the path to sublimation.

Thus both of them have no way of existing other than in this elsewhere; and it is symbolization which organizes the passage through this other place. That man is 'all' does not place him outside of the system of demand.

Neither man nor woman (nor a woman) can say: I am beauty; nor can they say: I am truth. But if, once, a word is said, it is because two voices meet there; and if a face appears, it is because beauty is assembled in it. Word spoken from one to the other; beauty of one contemplated by the other according to the separation of the sexes. The word is heard and beauty is seen, on condition that they are from one to the other, man or woman.

No face – on the other hand – is interposed in the analytic treatment. There is no case to answer. Thus the analysand is precipitated in fantasy. Françoise Dolto says that in analysis 'you spend your time failing to attract'. The analysand speaks, or keeps quiet; he tells dreams; and he even dreams with the sole aim of one day hearing this 'I fancy you'. But the 'I fancy you', turning the analysand into the object (a) of the analyst, would at the same time make the treatment fail. It is only when the fabric of fantasy, through lack of support, reveals the hole, that the analysand can turn around.

Woman, as the one who knows about the origin, and as the attendant to the function of (a), seems fated to take the place of the analyst, with the decisive difference that, sphinx, prostitute or mother, she does not bring about any subject from that place: 'You wanted to prostitute yourself, that's all you wanted to do,' said an analysand one day, to her analyst whom she thought too seductive. And if the analyst, like the prostitute, withdraws his face from the scene, it is not so much that he is without desire in this matter, but that his sole desire as analyst is to bring about the other as subject; not without risk for himself, since his own relation to the world is changed through it.

The analytic act is not undertaken – in opposition to the sexual act – on a gaze, even if it means blinding this gaze in order to find the sex. Bringing about the subject where the unconscious speaks implies there is no case to answer, the quite empty barrier, and not this solid screen made up of the meeting of two crossing gazes where a face would rise. If, at the end, the analysand discovers a face when turning around, he will go on discovering many others with the same surprise; and if he is a man, it may be a woman's face. The unavoidable alternative of the sexless face or the faceless sex may then eventually be resolved in an encounter.

Défilés: The pathways of desire, which has to go through demand; they are equally those of the signifying chain, having to go through the thresholds of a path full of solutions of continuity.

Demand: It is the metonymy of need on the one hand, and of desire on the other.

Desire: Desire of the Other and, because of it, never to find its object since there is no Other of the Other.

Discourse: In the Lacanian sense there are four discourses which are structures of four elements each: object (a), the barred subject $, Signifier 1 and Signifier 2.

Foreclosure: That which is foreclosed in the symbolic comes back in the real. The inaugural foreclosure, when it happens, is that of the Name-of-the-Father. If this inaugural metaphor doesn't take place, the signifying chain has not been constituted, and psychosis ensues.

Fort-Da: The childish game described by Freud which has become the paradigm of presence and absence. The young child throws a cotton reel and says 'Fort' ('Gone'); when the reel is retrieved, the child says 'Da' ('There'). The game is played again and again in an effort to come to terms psychically with the mother's comings and goings.

Hysteria: Characterized by the appeal to the Other, who is supposed to carry the phallus. It is the only one amongst the nosographic entities to found a discourse.

The Imaginary: For Lacan, the human function closest to the animal world. It is the faculty of responding to a similar form. It is constitutive of the species, and fuels the illusion of sameness.

Lack: What is lacking in order for there to be a whole.

Lack of Being: What being lacks in order to be a self-sufficient All-Being; also a moment of the end of analysis, when the object (a), this plug-on lack, detaches itself.

Lure: The function of **lure** is that of the object (a); it causes desire without being constituted as its object; and it is the object of the drive, only to slide away from its grasp. It is only a starting mechanism, allowing the libidinal apparatus to function.

Méconnaissance: Repression may come with **méconnaissance** if the subject persists in not wanting to know, in refusing to recognize wishes and desires.

Metaphor: Result of a process in which a thing is put in the place of another; thus transference is a particular case of metaphor; so is 'condensation' in its Freudian sense; and so is language, since the word is put in the place of the thing.

Metonymy: As the signifier does not exhaust the signified, signification can be said to be the consequence of a metaphorico-metonymic sequence. Lacan linked metonymy to the connection of word-to-word, and related this to the Freudian 'displacement'.

Need: Demands satisfaction; it is instinctual.

Object (a): The object as cause of desire. Thus it is not strictly an object; nor, in any case, the object of desire. It is the object of the drive; but the drive only goes around it, it does not reach

it. There are four objects (a): the breast, the faeces, the gaze and the voice.

Other: The great Other. But there is no Other of the Other. That is to say, there is no being which could constitute absolute otherness for a subject.

Phallic Function: Written (φx) in the Lacanian texts. (φx) is the feature which characterizes humans, gathered into a whole because of it, on the condition that there be at least one of them to say no to the phallic function. The phallic function consists in raising the penis to the dignity of the phallus with a gain and a loss.

Phallic Jouissance: The **jouissance** of the Other as such; that is to say as other. The object (a) and the great Other are joined in it. It is the **jouissance** of the speaking being.

The Real: That which man – the being of language – separates himself from, and, in so doing, names.

Real, Imaginary, Symbolic: These can only be defined in relation to one another. This ternary relation is substituted by Lacan for the binary relation: form/content; imaginary/ real; symbol/being. The imaginary and the symbolic become knotted in the real, as a Borromean knot shows (but doesn't demonstrate) in the very making of the knot.

Signified: The signifier has a signified; this is written: $\frac{S}{s}$. This 's' which is the signified designates the subject as well. In any case the algorithm $\frac{S}{s}$ signifies that the signifier comes in the place of the signified. But it does not exhaust it; there is always a left over: x.

Signifier: That which represents a subject for another signifier. One cannot stress enough that it does not concern a simple, entirely linear chain of signifiers, as for instance: S, S1, S2 . . . . S^n.

Specular Image: Lacan writes that from the age of six months, the child can recognize himself in a mirror and is jubilant at the time of this recognition. This experience of the unifying orthopedic specular image is also deceiving, and opens up the so-called mirror stage.

Supplementary Jouissance: The *jouissance* of the Other, without the object (a) being implicated in it.

The Symbolic: Taken separately, the symbolic is the category of language, regardless of the material of language (words, dreams, gestures, etc.).

Symbolic Castration: In opposition to real castration (ablation of the penis) and to imaginary castration (neurotic impotence). It is also in opposition to deprivation, which is real, and to frustration, which is imaginary. Symbolic castration is the consequence of a function of language which ratifies the impossibility of the sexual relation, but which does not deny sexual desire at work in the unconscious structured like a language.

BIBLIOGRAPHY

Aeschylus, *The Eumenides* in D. Grene and R. Lattimore, eds *The Complete Greek Tragedies*, vol. 1. Chicago: University of Chicago Press, 1953.

Ancelet-Hustache, J. (1976) *Goethe par lui-même*. Paris: Le Seuil.

Anon. (1952) La secte des Anandrynes. Paris: Briffault.

Apollinaire, G. (1946) *Les mamelles de Tirésias*. Paris: Gallimard, 1972.

Barnes, M. and Berke, J. (1971) *Mary Barnes: Two Accounts of a Journey through Madness*. London: Penguin Books.

Bataille, G. (1966) *The Mother*. London: Jonathan Cape, 1978.

—(1973) *Théorie de la religion*. Paris: Gallimard.

Bateson, G. (1961) *Percival's Narrative, a Patient's Account of his Psychosis*. Stanford, CA: Stanford University Press.

Binswanger, L. (1944) 'The case of Ellen West', in R. May, ed. *Existence, a new Dimension in Psychiatry and Psychology*. New York: Basic, 1958.

Cardinal, M. (1973) *The Words To Say It*, P. Goodheart, trans. London: Picador, 1983.

Chardin, B. (1974) 'Problèmes de la grossesse pendant la cure', *Le Coq Héron* 36.

Chesler, P. (1972) *Women and Madness*. New York: Doubleday.

Cixous, H. (1975) *L'Arc* 61.

Cixous, H. and Clément, C. (1975) *The Newly Born Woman*. Manchester: Manchester University Press, 1986.

Delcourt, M. (1958) *Hermaphrodite, mythes et rites de la bisexualité dans la Grèce antique*. Paris: Presses

Universitaires de France.

Deleuze, G. (1969) *La logique du sens*. Paris: Editions de Minuit.

Djedidi, T.L. (1974) *La poésie amoureuse des Arabes*. Algiers: SNED.

Duras, M. and Gauthier, X. (1974) *Les parleuses*. Paris: Editions de Minuit.

Ebtinger, R. and Renoux, M. (1967) 'Aspects psycho-pathologiques de la paternité', *Lettres de l'Ecole Freudienne* 4.

Eliade, M. (1962) *Méphistophélès et l'androgyne*. Paris: Gallimard.

Ellis, H. (1951) *Sex and Marriage: Eros in Contemporary Life*. London: Greenwood Press, 1977.

Faulkner, W. (1932) *Light in August*. London: Penguin Books, 1985.

Fernandez, D. (1974) *Porporino*. Paris: Grasset.

Freud, S. (1908) 'Hysterical phantasies and their relation to bisexuality', in James Strachey, ed. *The Standard Edition of the Complete Psychological Works of Sigmund Freud*, 24 vols. London: Hogarth, 1953-73. vol. 9, pp. 157-66.

—(1912) 'On the universal tendency to debasement in the sphere of love'. *S.E.* 11, pp. 179-90.

—(1914) 'On narcissism, an introduction'. *S.E.* 14, pp. 73-102.

—(1917) 'On transformations of instinct as exemplified in anal eroticism'. *S.E.* 17, pp. 127-33.

—(1931) 'Female sexuality'. *S.E.* 21, pp. 225-43.

Genet, J. (1962) *The Balcony*, B. Frechtman, trans. London: Faber & Faber, 1957.

Gide, A. (1920) *Corydon*. London: Farrar, Strauss & Giroux, 1983.

Goethe, J.W. von (1776) *Die Geschwister*, in *Dramatische Dichtungen*, 2. München: Beck, 1982.

—(1809) *Elective Affinities*, R. J. Hollingdale, trans. London: Penguin Books, 1971.

—(1829a) *Wilhelm Meister's Years of Travel or the Renunciants*, H.M. Waidson, trans. London: Jonathan Calder, 1980.

—(1829) *The Man of Fifty*, H. M. Waidson, trans. London: Jonathan Calder, 1980.

—(1907) *Maximen und Reflexionen*. Weimar: Verlag der Goethe Gesellschaft.

Granoff, W. and Périer, F. (1964) 'Recherches sur la féminité', *La Psychanalyse* 7. Paris: Presses Universitaires de France.

Guir, J. (1975-6) 'Exposé sur Fliess'. Contribution to Seminar, 'Féminité, grossesse et sexualité'.

Hassoun, J. (1975) 'La plainte des femmes'. *Lettres de l'Ecole Freudienne* 17.

Hegel, G.W.F. (1905) *Phenomenology of Spirit*, A.V. Miller, trans. Oxford: Oxford University Press, 1977.

Hoffmansthal, H. von (1919) *Die Frau ohne Schatten*. Berlin.

Irigaray, L. (1974a) *The Speculum of the Other Woman*, G.C. Gill, trans. Ithaca, NY: Cornell University Press, 1985.

—(1974b) 'La tache aveugle dans un vieux rêve de symétrie', *Critique* 278.

Jakobson, R. (1942) 'Kindersprache, Aphasie und allgemeine Lautgesetze', in *Selected Writings I*. The Hague: Mouton, 1962.

Kerenyi, C. (1967) *Eleusis*. New York: Pantheon Books.

Lacan, J. (1956-7) *Le séminaire III: les psychoses*. Paris: Editions du Seuil, 1981.

—(1960) *Le séminaire VII: l'éthique*. Paris: Editions du Seuil.

—(1964) *The Four Fundamental Concepts of Psycho-Analysis*. London: Penguin Books, 1979.

—(1966) *Ecrits*. London: Tavistock Publications, 1977.

—(1972-3) *Le séminaire XX: Encore*. Paris: Editions du Seuil, 1975.

—(1973) *De la psychose paranoïaque dans ses rapports avec la personnalité*. Paris: Editions du Seuil.

—(1974-5) *Le séminaire: RSI*. Paris: Editions du Seuil.

Lacoue-Labarthe, P. (1975) 'L'imprésentable', *Poétique* 21: 53-95.

Legendre, P. (1974) *L'amour du censeur*. Paris: Editions du Seuil.

Lemoine, G. and Lemoine, P. (1972) *Le psychodrame.* Paris: Laffont.

Lemoine, P. (1974) Contribution to Seminar, 'Féminité, grossesse, sexualité'.

Lévi-Strauss, C. (1962) *The Savage Mind.* University of Chicago Press, 1968.

—(1971) *The Naked Man*, J. and D. Weightman, trans. London: Jonathan Cape, 1981.

Lombroso, G. (1924) *L'âme de la femme.* Paris: Payot.

Luccioni, G. (1959) 'La méthode de Musil', *Esprit.*

Luccioni, M. (1976) *Wie nu geen huis heeft.*

Maillet, C. (1974) Contribution to Seminar, 'Féminité, grossesse et sexualité'.

—(1975) *Lettres de l'Ecole Freudienne* 14.

Mann, K. (1936) *Mephisto: Roman einer Karriere.* Reinbeck bei Hamburg: Rowohlt Taschenbuch Verlag, 1981.

Mann, T. (1905) 'The blood of the Walsungs', in *Stories of Three Decades*, H.T. Lowe-Porter, trans. New York: Alfred A. Knopf, 1936.

—(1951) *The Holy Sinner*, H.T. Lowe-Porter, trans. London: Penguin Books, 1975.

Mintz, I.L. (1975) 'Parapraxis and the mother-child relationship', *Psychoanal. Q.* 3.

Monesi, I. (1966) *Nature morte devant la fenêtre.* Paris: Mercure de France.

Montrelay, M. (1970) 'Recherches sur la féminité', *Critique.*

Musil, R. (1930) *The Man without Qualities*, E. Wilkins and E. Kaiser, trans. London: Picador, 1979.

Nasio, J.D. and Taillandier, G. (n.d.) 'Gorgonéion' (unpublished).

Niedermann, W.G. (1975) *Psychoanal. Q.* 3.

Obaldia, R. de (1975) 'Monsieur Klebs et Rosalie', in *Théâtre VI.* Paris: Grasset.

Paulhan, J. (1953) *La preuve par l'étymologie.* Paris: Editions de Minuit.

Pécaut, M. (1974-5) Contribution to Seminar, 'Féminité, grossesse et sexualité'.

Ramnoux, C. (1974) *Revue de métaphysique et morale.* Paris: Armand Colin.

Rank, O. (1932) *Don Juan: une étude sur le double*. Paris: Payot, 1973.

Réage, P. (1954) *The Story of O*, S. Estree, trans. London: Corgi, 1972.

Reik, T. (1946) *The Ritual*. New York: International Universities Press, 1976.

Rezvani, C. (1976) *Le portrait ovale*. Paris: Gallimard.

Righini, M. (1975) 'Enquête sur le suicide', *Le Nouvel Observateur* 554.

Rotter, L. (1932) *Revue française de psychanalyse*, I. Barande, trans. 1975.

Roubin, L.A. (1970) *Les chambrettes des Provençaux*. Paris: Plon.

Rouy, C. (1974) Contribution to Seminar, 'Féminité, grossesse, sexualité'.

Santos, E. (1973) *La malcastrée*. Paris: Maspéro.

Schreber, D.P. (1903) *Memoirs of my Nervous Illness*, I. Macalpine and R.A. Hunter, trans. London: William Dawson & Sons, 1955. *Mémoires d'un névropathe*, N. Sels and P. Duquenne, trans. Paris: Editions du Seuil, 1975.

Scilicet 4 (1973) 'Le meurtre de l'enfant'.

This, B. (1975) 'Le placenta', *Lettres de l'Ecole Freudienne* 14.

Tolstoy, L. (1889) *The Kreutzer Sonata*, in *The Kreutzer Sonata and Other Stories*. London: Penguin Books, 1985.

Tournier, M. (1967) *Friday or the Other Island*, Norman Denny, trans. London: Methuen, 1969.

—(1970) *The Erl-King*, B. Bray, trans. London: Methuen, 1983.

—(1975) *Gemini*. London: Methuen, 1985.

Valéry, P. (1917) *La jeune Parque*. Paris: Edisud, 1982.

Weininger, O. (1906) *On the Character of Man*. New Atlantic Foundation, 1982.

Wolff, C. (1971) *Love between Women*. London: Duckworth, 1973.

INDEX

This first English edition of
THE DIVIDING OF WOMEN or WOMAN'S LOT
was finished in September 1987.

It was phototypeset in 10½/14 pt Bodoni
on a Linotron 202 and printed by
a Heidelberg SORS offset press
on 80g/m² vol. 18 Supreme Antique Wove.

The translation was commissioned by Robert M. Young,
edited by Ann Scott, copy-edited by Sara Beardsworth,
indexed by Fiona Barr, designed by Carlos Sapochnik
and produced by David Williams and Selina O'Grady
for Free Association Books.